Overcoming Acute
and Chronic Pain

"*Overcoming Acute and Chronic Pain* is one of the best books in its field to emerge in recent years. It breaks new ground—choosing a pain therapy based not just on one's medical diagnosis but also on one's emotional patterns. As Micozzi and Dibra show, this approach can have an enormous impact on a therapy's effectiveness. If you or a loved one suffers from acute or chronic pain, or if you are a medical professional who deals with such, please pay attention to the wisdom of this important book."

LARRY DOSSEY, M.D., AUTHOR OF
ONE MIND: HOW OUR INDIVIDUAL MIND IS PART OF
A GREATER CONSCIOUSNESS AND WHY IT MATTERS

"This book is full of well-researched solutions that are helpful, healing, non-addicting, and get to the core of the issue, creating better health and relief for those that implement these time-tested solutions."

BRIGITTE MARS, AUTHOR OF
ADDICTION-FREE NATURALLY AND THE SEXUAL HERBAL

PRAISE FOR
YOUR EMOTIONAL TYPE
by Marc S. Micozzi, M.D., Ph.D.,
and Michael A. Jawer

"The book is empowering, helping us to become active agents in our healing rather than being simply the recipients of 'cures' from a medical approach that fails to recognize the uniqueness of individuals."

GABOR MATÉ, M.D., AUTHOR OF *WHEN THE BODY SAYS NO: EXPLORING THE STRESS-DISEASE CONNECTION*

". . . offers a valuable framework for helping people choose among the array of complementary and alternative therapies."

DEANE JUHAN, AUTHOR OF
JOB'S BODY: A HANDBOOK FOR BODYWORK

"*Your Emotional Type* is a wake-up call for those who are stuck in stubborn emotional prisons of fear, anger, resentment, regret, and self-destruction."

SPIRITUALITY & PRACTICE

Overcoming Acute
and Chronic Pain

Keys to Treatment Based on
Your Emotional Type

Marc S. Micozzi, M.D., Ph.D.,
and
Sebhia Marie Dibra

Healing Arts Press
Rochester, Vermont • Toronto, Canada

Healing Arts Press
One Park Street
Rochester, Vermont 05767
www.healingArtsPress.com

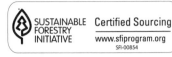

Text stock is SFI certified

Healing Arts Press is a division of Inner Traditions International

Note to the reader: This book is intended as an informational guide. The remedies, approaches, and techniques described herein are meant to supplement, and not to be a substitute for, professional medical care or treatment. They should not be used to treat a serious ailment without prior consultation with a qualified health care professional.

Library of Congress Cataloging-in-Publication Data

Names: Micozzi, Marc S., 1953- author. | Dibra, Sebhia M., 1988- author.

Title: Overcoming acute and chronic pain : keys to treatment based on your emotional type / Marc S. Micozzi, M.D., Ph.D., and Sebhia M. Dibra.

Description: Rochester, Vermont : Healing Arts Press, [2017] | Includes bibliographical references and index.

Identifiers: LCCN 2016018706 (print) | LCCN 2016023782 (e-book) | ISBN 9781620555637 (paperback) | ISBN 9781620555644 (e-book)

Subjects: LCSH: Pain—Alternative treatment. | Medicine, Psychosomatic. | Alternative medicine. | BISAC: HEALTH & FITNESS / Alternative Therapies. | HEALTH & FITNESS / Pain Management. | MEDICAL / Holistic Medicine.

Classification: LCC RB127 .M53 2017 (print) | LCC RB127 (e-book) | DDC 616/.0472—dc23

LC record available at https://lccn.loc.gov/2016018706

Printed and bound in the United States by Lake Book Manufacturing, Inc. The text stock is SFI certified. The Sustainable Forestry Initiative® program promotes sustainable forest management.

10 9 8 7 6 5 4 3 2 1

Text design by Debbie Glogover and layout by Virginia Scott Bowman
This book was typeset in Garamond Premier Pro, Gill Sans, Futura, and Agenda with Else NPL and Futura used as display typefaces

To send correspondence to the authors of this book, mail a first-class letter to the authors c/o Inner Traditions • Bear & Company, One Park Street, Rochester, VT 05767, and we will forward the communication, or contact the authors directly at **www.drmicozzi.com** or **www.sebhiadibra.com**.

Contents

PART TWO

Hands-On Healing

PART THREE

Managing Pain with Natural Products

Acknowledgments

Marc Micozzi would like to acknowledge his colleague Michael Jawer for his years of work applying the personality boundary and emotional psychometric types to the various mind-body conditions considered in this book, as well as in previous books that we coauthored: *Spiritual Anatomy of Emotion* and *Your Emotional Type*.

In addition, both authors wish to acknowledge Denise Rodgers for her early original insights into many of the connections and continuities among various mind-body therapies; Marty Rossman for his pioneering work, case histories, and contributions over many years to the field and practice of guided imagery therapy; and the late David Larson for his original work and promotion of the study of prayer, religious practice, and spirituality in healing. We are grateful to Dan Redwood for his decades of work in education and research on spinal manual therapy and chiropractic and to Judith Walker Delany for her contributions to massage as a medical therapy and health and wellness practice. We give special recognition to Kevin Ergil and Marnae Ergil for their unique and comprehensive knowledge, perspectives, and contributions in classical Chinese medicine and acupuncture and to Caroline Hoffman and Rhiannon Lewis for their steadfast work, contributions, teachings, and overall leadership on the health benefits of aromatherapy and essential oils therapy. We acknowledge science journalist Charles Seife for his explanation of the principles of matter and antimatter that embody the infinite universe, as well as the neuroscientists at the University of Oxford, England, for their significant contributions to the neuroscience community. In early 2015, these Oxford researchers discovered the location of a "pain center" in the brain that becomes active based on how much pain a person perceives.

Thank you to our editors at Inner Traditions, Meghan MacLean and Margaret Jones, for going above and beyond. And thank you to Jon Graham and Ehud Sperling for having faith in our continued vision for helping people by using the emotional boundary types.

Finally, we acknowledge the team of gifted young writers and editors at Omni Vista Health for assistance in keeping up with all the latest, groundbreaking scientific developments that offer promising, innovative natural approaches for pain.

Taking a
Natural Approach to Pain

While most of the mind-body pain disorders addressed in this book are poorly understood and poorly treated by Western medical care, they account for a huge amount of daily distress, discomfort, and disability. And these conditions are often chronic. Chronic diseases are those that are prolonged, do not resolve spontaneously, and are rarely cured completely. The rarity of complete cures in conventional medicine is related to the incompleteness of the old twentieth-century medical model of disease.

In 2003 the Centers for Disease Control and Prevention (CDC) announced that chronic diseases affect almost 100 million Americans and account for one-third of the years of potential life lost before the age of sixty-five. The financial burden of treating chronic diseases now accounts for almost two-thirds of the total medical care costs in the United States.

Complementary and alternative (or integrative) medicine, or CAM, defines a broad category of interventions, such as the mind-body modalities described in this book, that have not been taught widely at U.S. medical schools or generally available at U.S. hospitals. Nevertheless, in the twenty-first century, almost half of the adult population in the United States is already using CAM to help manage chronic diseases.

There has been growing awareness in recent years that one of the major motivations for learning, seeking, and applying what has been called "natural medicine," which we see as synonymous with CAM, is to address the prodigious problem of pain. In fact, the medical textbook *Fundamentals of Complementary and Alternative Medicine* (now in its sixth edition), written and edited by half of this author team, Marc Micozzi, has been the most requested book at the annual meetings of the American Association for Pain Management, although this basic text is a foundational survey of CAM approaches for health care professionals and is not especially focused on pain. This new book for health care consumers attempts to do just that; it has been written on the basis of information available from a multitude of medical and scientific literature, with the consumer foremost in mind. The dimensions and parameters of the pain problem have expanded dramatically over the past twenty years because of the aging population that is facing new challenges with respect to pain, including the looming use, misuse, and abuse of both legal pain medications and illegal drugs. The overwhelming implications for public health, law enforcement, and public policy have become evident across the county and worldwide. In my (Micozzi speaking here) former practice of forensic medicine, I encountered many cases of death from drug overdose (usually pain drugs). These overdoses were intentional (suicide), accidental, and occasionally homicidal. From an insurance standpoint, the main concern was determining not the manner of death, but whether the levels of drugs detected were consistent with the prescribed dosages.

Meanwhile, there have been large shifts in the accepted paradigm for health and healing when it comes to elucidating and understanding the bioenergetic model and the consciousness dimension of human health. In some places, medical practice is incorporating CAM under the rubric of so-called integrative medicine. In terms of this integration, the patient is confronted with a bewildering array of different ,CAM therapies from over twenty different major healing traditions, ranging from single, simple techniques to entire systems of medical practice and health care. *Overcoming Acute and Chronic Pain: Keys to Treatment Based on Your Emotional Type* is a guide for navigating the CAM waters, with specific guidance for you personally as an individual.

This book is personalized for you because it includes a time-tested, easy-to-use psychometric evaluation that associates the susceptibility of different persons to chronic medical conditions and treatments—a premise originally presented in Mike Jawer and Marc Micozzi's 2011 book *Your Emotional Type*. Understanding your emotional type through this personalized assessment shows you which CAM therapies will best work for you, and which conditions are best treated by specific CAM therapies. From among the many different CAM options there are many safe and effective alternatives to prescription drugs for treating pain. Nature's original pain medication from the opium poppy—morphine, named after the Greek god of sleep, Morpheus—has been supplanted by synthetic or semisynthetic prescription drugs (e.g., Fentanyl) and illegal drugs (e.g., di-acetyl morphine, or heroin), some of which are many times more powerful than what can be found anywhere in nature. The development of drug approaches to both pain and to pain-drug addiction and dependence has led to its own industry and social institutions, as found in the network of methadone clinics, which themselves have spawned additional problems for medicine and public health and safety.

In recent years, both mind-body CAM approaches as well as vitamins, nutritional foods, herbs, and essential oils have undergone scientific research for their application in pain management, and these are described in this book for you, the health care consumer. Natural approaches generally, and herbal medicine specifically, are typically less potent (and thus safer) than prescription pain medications. But there are examples when the appropriate micronutrient doses of herbal remedies are actually more effective compared to the standard drug treatments for certain pain conditions. Some long-standing prescription drugs (e.g., Darvon) and over-the-counter drugs (e.g., acetaminophen, trade name Tylenol) have also been shown to be completely ineffective for common pain conditions—and their significant toxicities must also be mentioned.

The drug-oriented approach to pain management is now being challenged due to its insurmountable problems and the emerging perspective on bioenergy and consciousness, which offers a new frontier for noninvasive pain management. These innovative nondrug approaches have become a focus of current medical observations as well as newer findings in the basic sciences and neurophysiology. In the context of this new and expanded view, the term *conscious pain and suffering,* which is typically used for medical-legal analysis in forensic medicine, proceedings, and jurisprudence, may be seen more broadly as *consciousness of* pain and suffering. A consciousness approach to pain and pain treatment is emphasized throughout this book.

Down through the ages, students and scholars of technological developments in human societies have often observed that the discovery of innovative ideas and approaches long precedes their widespread acceptance and application, supplanting older, less effective practices. Usually the old approaches and practices are not replaced with the "better idea" until people are overwhelmed with problems that threaten society as a whole. Such is the time we are in right now when it comes to drug approaches to pain. The time may be right to finally improve on the old approach and all its concurrent medical and social problems.

Fortunately, CAM offers us a new world of opportunities for nondrug pain treatments that are time-tested and increasingly being substantiated by new discoveries in modern clinical trials. This book provides the background and science to support the use of CAM and natural approaches in cases of acute and chronic pain, individualized for you, the health care consumer.

The Problem of Pain

We have over forty years of combined experience investigating and researching nondrug, natural treatments for pain, inflammation, and pain-related conditions, and new research confirming these approaches is growing exponentially. Every time we write something on the topic, more research comes in before the ink is dry. Complementary and mind-body therapies in general have many applications in addressing functional complaints, such as pain, and chronic pain disorders.

Pain and headache (head pain) are perhaps the two most common functional disorders of the human condition, experienced by virtually everyone on an acute basis at one time or another, and by millions on a chronic, episodic, or recurring basis. Throughout history, much of the effort in human healing traditions has been directed at analgesia—the alleviation of pain—through the discovery and development of materia medica (opiates, salicylates, etc.), physical manipulation (e.g., bone setting, chiropractic, traditional osteopathy, physical therapy), and massage, yoga, acupuncture, and mind-body approaches, all of which are addressed in this book. Energy healing represents a new frontier, yet it has ancient roots.

In the early history of American medicine, alleviating pain, together with preventing death, was one of the two central tenets of "rational medicine." Rational medicine in practice was a result of the eighteenth-century Scottish Enlightenment, which was characterized by an outpouring of intellectual and scientific accomplishments as manifested in the field of economics by social philosopher Adam Smith, for example. In the mid-1700s it was brought to what was then known as the "American colonies" by doctors Morgan and Hutchinson of the University of Edinburgh, to the College of Philadelphia (now the University of Pennsylvania); there, the first school of medicine in what was to later become the United States was established in 1765 by charter from colonial governor John Penn. The rest is American medical history.

Today, pain is understood as a dynamic condition, not a static pathological state or defect. And while curing or removing a painful lesion may eliminate the pain (with the curious exception of conditions such as phantom-limb syndrome experienced by amputees), pain exists in many other contexts where there is no identifiable defect or abnormality to cure or remove.

Therefore, the assessment and management of pain, whether alternative or mainstream, must lie in the interaction between the mind and the body, the healer and the patient, and the patient and the therapy.

Pain is a subjective complaint, and therefore its improvement is also subjective, yet associated with very high levels of patient satisfaction. Mind-body approaches are proving successful in the management of pain. The seventeenth-century Cartesian principle of the separation of mind and body has been an artificial accommodation to the philosophically limited understanding of health and healing that has prevailed for so long. This outdated concept of separation, which continues in Western medicine (but is not a factor in ancient Asian medical traditions, as we shall see later in this book), perhaps influences how we are conditioned to experience and express pain. In traditional societies in Africa and elsewhere, as an example, psychic pain is often "somatized" to a specific area of the body and presents as pain in a particular body part rather than as a general mental state.

The entire body acts beyond the brain-body barrier as an organ of consciousness through the movements of "molecules of emotion," a theory postulated by the late neuroscientist Candace Pert. In this scenario, mind-body distinctions begin to lose their meaning. A "gut feeling" is really being felt in the gut. And some of the diffuse pain associated with chronic fatigue syndrome and fibromyalgia, for example, may ultimately be a conditioned response emanating from elsewhere.

The successful alleviation of pain and the treatment of other neurological conditions can no longer be considered alternative versus mainstream. What works should simply be considered good medicine.

YOUR PROBLEM, YOUR PAIN

Pain is the problem most commonly reported to doctors. Patients with chronic pain and other neurological conditions feel helpless and frustrated. The events and stories surrounding their suffering are innumerable and continue to pose challenges for all those concerned with human health and wellness.

Science and medicine have made remarkable progress in many realms. Mortality rates have long been in decline, and people have been living longer, but with some alarming recent exceptions in some populations that have experienced dramatically *increased* death rates over the past fifteen years, due primarily to use and abuse of pain drugs. This has resulted in changes in disease patterns and patient priorities. Chronic diseases such as arthritis, musculoskeletal pain, mental-health problems, and neurological conditions such as Alzheimer's and stroke are becoming more common. Those who suffer continue to live and look for ways and means to alleviate their pain and agony.

Modern medicine views the human body as a biomedical machine that can be analyzed and, when needed, repaired, altered, or modified structurally. Surgery remains a very effective treatment for most acute traumatic injuries. The skills of modern mainstream health practitioners in treating acute emergency illnesses remain unsurpassed. However, the current high technology–based health care system is not without many limitations and problems when it comes to addressing acute and chronic pain. While the modern health care system is generally effective in managing most infectious diseases, traumatic injuries, and other acute problems, it is limited in helping those with chronic diseases and the resulting pain, the causes of which are related to a number of factors. Modern chronic-pain treatments such as surgery and pain medications, for example, are inadequate for many, and in many instances are not safe. Those using pain drugs combined with other medications run a risk for developing some serious problems. Pain drugs are now recognized as one of today's major public safety and public health problems.

For this reason, approaches that encourage people to participate in their own personalized healing and that offer natural, complementary and alternative medicine (CAM) treatments are gaining in popularity worldwide. Such approaches are producing positive results scientifically as well as forming the basis of a refreshing, innovative, integrative method of treatment and healing. Since it is now well known that not all alternative therapies work equally well for all people with pain, the new frontier is in helping pain sufferers find the right treatments that will work best for them. Our work on the psychometrics of personality boundary types and emotional types, as delineated in chapter 1, gives you the tools you need to find out which pain treatments will work best for you and your condition.

Evidence from recent scientific studies shows both the usefulness and the limitations associated with various treatments. There is sufficient evidence, for example, to support the use of acupuncture for chronic low-back pain and dental pain; hypnosis for pain and anxiety; and mind-body techniques such as meditation, yoga, and biofeedback for chronic pain. Doctors who utilize these therapies in their practices report benefits for both their patients and themselves. There are many CAM therapies, however, that have yet to routinely show benefits for all people, and some that might present an unjustifiable risk (for example, coffee enemas, Laetrile, ozone therapy, and megadoses of vitamins and shark cartilage). Use of these unproven or disproven therapies may also result in the loss of valuable time and the opportunity to receive potentially beneficial therapies. But even for the commonly available and proven pain remedies presented in this book, we still need to apply ways to match the best treatment for each individual person who suffers from pain. This book presents an approach that you can begin using today to find out which of these alternative pain remedies will work best for you, and why.

THE COMPLEXITY OF TREATING PAIN

Where you live might actually determine the level of pain-management care you receive. A recent report on the treatment of pain in the United States shows that thirty-five states don't adequately address the issue, which means pain is a major public-health challenge for the remaining states.[1] Alabama, Idaho, Georgia, Iowa, Kansas, Maine, Massachusetts, Michigan, Montana, Oregon, Rhode Island, and Vermont all earn high marks for being places with more balanced approaches to pain care that integrate CAM therapies. California, Washington D.C., Hawaii, Illinois, Maryland, Minnesota, New York, and Washington State—all places with big state and local governments and health departments where one might expect better health care—are all oddly missing from this list of having good approaches to pain care.

Pain is often a symptom of other medical problems; for example, one-third of cancer patients suffer from chronic pain as a result of their cancer and/or the standard medical treatment of it. But pain is also a complex problem in its own right. It can actually change the nervous system and become its own distinct, chronic disease. According to the European Association for Palliative Care, one-third of patients with chronic pain report that it's so bad they have wanted to die.[2]

Older Americans face a disproportionate burden of pain. A 2010 study found that between 25 and 40 percent of men and women over the age of sixty-five suffer from pain daily.[3] Plus, the proportion of patients adequately medicated for pain actually decreases with increasing age. In other words, the older you get, the less effectively your pain is treated. To compound matters, men and women with cognitive impairment, such as Alzheimer's and dementia, often can't even report their own pain effectively.

Many veterans also suffer from chronic pain. In a June 2014 study published in the *Journal of the American Medical Association,* researchers followed 2,500 soldiers recently returned from combat deployment; 44 percent of the soldiers had chronic pain, and 15 percent of them used narcotic pain relievers to deal with it—a percentage much higher than in the general population.[4]

Mainstream medicine focuses only on the visible and the objective, so it seeks to find simple, generic solutions to complex problems. But pain doesn't work that way. It's highly individual and subjective. Plus, it's based on constitutional factors and/or sociocultural factors. Most importantly, pain is not just a physical problem; there are profound mental dimensions to it. Studies on veterans have found a strong association between chronic pain and suicide. These findings were consistent with the findings of the European Association for Palliative Care.

In sum, physicians simply are not trained thoroughly on pain and pain identification (though Big Pharma makes sure physicians get plenty of training on prescribing drugs). On average, a physician receives just eight hours of training on how to treat pain. By comparison, a veterinarian receives eighty-seven hours of training on how to treat pain in animals.

Make no mistake, prescription painkillers can be a viable short-term treatment choice, particularly after major surgery or dental work. But the use of prescription pain drugs is fraught with peril. First, the government's counterproductive war on drugs allows the DEA to interfere with how physicians treat their patients, and that interference goes even beyond the usual kind run by the FDA. Second, doctors feel intimidated about prescribing (and nurses feel reluctant to administer) adequate pain medication, even to those dying and in pain from terminal conditions. Third, these drugs *do* have high potential for addiction. And they're dangerous. The CDC reports that forty-six Americans die every day from prescription painkillers.

As with other medical conditions, chronic pain has repercussions that go far beyond any simple drug. Fortunately, many natural mind-body approaches can help control pain and improve quality of life. Yet the average physician knows nothing about these effective nondrug treatments. People respond remarkably differently to nondrug therapies, just as they do to drugs. For example, many people benefit from massage. Others benefit more from low-impact exercise such as swimming, walking, or stationary bicycling. More formal approaches include yoga and tai chi. You also need to get good sleep to manage pain. Counseling and physical therapy can help as well. Unfortunately, there's no single silver bullet for managing pain.

RECENT SCIENTIFIC EVIDENCE

A good example of an approach that relies on the power of the mind to help manage pain is guided imagery, in which you are guided by a professional to form images in your "mind's eye" that help you to literally overcome your pain. One of the most common, and problematic, orthopedic surgical procedures today is knee replacement, ostensibly done to reduce pain and improve function of the knee (although researchers have found two-thirds of these surgeries are inappropriate).[5] Guided imagery is now being recommended as a natural therapy for pain relief following orthopedic knee-replacement surgery. New research shows that guided imagery is a useful treatment for most patients, and they show high levels of participation and satisfaction when offered this therapy for pain following surgery.[6]

Another natural mind-body powerhouse for addressing pain is mindfulness meditation along with mindfulness-based stress reduction (MBSR). A 2015 study demonstrated that MBSR was effective in reducing pain and improving the quality of life in patients with chronic low-back pain after only eight sessions (the standard approach to group MBSR).[7] Of course, anxiety and depression often accompany chronic pain. In another 2015 study, a group of chronic-pain patients who completed a mindfulness-meditation training program demonstrated significant improvement in anxiety, depression, and pain over a one-year observation period.[8] The standard MBSR program, which is evaluated in research studies, consists of eight weekly sessions. But you can gain many of the benefits of meditation in your daily life without signing up for formal classes (or without entering a Buddhist monastery).

Powerful and proven ancient herbal remedies are also available for pain and inflammation, especially for joint pain; we call them "the ABCs": ashwagandha, boswellia, and curcumin (see chapter 11 for more information on these). These three pain powerhouses have gained increasing scientific attention not only for their success in treating pain and inflammation, but for a host of other health benefits for brain and body.

One new study looked at use of a boswellia extract compared to standard medical treatment for the management of knee osteoarthritis symptoms. Compared to standard medical treatment, those given boswellia had just as good a reduction of pain and restoration of function, better overall emotional and social functions, and better overall physical performance as those treated with pharmaceutical drugs.[9]

Curcumin, a compound found in turmeric, is effective in addressing a wide range of inflammatory conditions. A new laboratory study used a novel approach—loading lipid (fat) nanoparticles into a curcumin supplement to treat rheumatoid arthritis. Results showed markedly improved levels of pain and molecular measures of inflammation.[10] Another 2014 study on a curcumin extract in a large general population of patients with osteoarthritis showed that subjects had improvements in pain, mobility, and quality of life within the first six weeks, and more than half of them were able to discontinue drugs for pain and inflammation.[11]

Of course, we have long observed that the ABCs are even more potent when taken together. A 2015 clinical trial study gave boswellia and curcumin together to patients following highly painful tendon repair, comparing it to standard drug treatment. The boswellia-curcumin combined treatment alleviated short-term and midterm pain better than drugs alone, but not long-term pain, for which researchers advised increasing the dosage of the herbs over the first four weeks and extending treatment by one to two months.[12]

And fish oil (taken essentially in food quantities) is a well-known anti-inflammatory. Two new major clinical trials of fish oil for the treatment of knee osteoarthritis showed benefits in improving knee performance.[13] And those benefits are just as good with a lower dose compared to a higher dose of fish oil.[14]

These are only a few of the very latest research developments on a wide variety of natural approaches to pain using mind-body practices, hands-on approaches, and natural products such as foods, herbs, dietary supplements, and plant essential oils. All of these subjects are covered in the the following chapters of this book.

PART ONE

≍+≍

Mind-Body Techniques
for Pain

1

Pain and
Your Emotional Type

The current epidemic of prescription pain-medication use and abuse in the United States has led to government calls for reducing our dependence on them, as well as for reducing the hazard of abuse of these narcotics. In 2015, after a century of improving health and declining death rates among women in this country, the Urban Institute released a study showing dramatically increasing death rates among women, due primarily to the increase in the use of these dangerous narcotic pain drugs. Perhaps even more shocking is data from the National Academy of Sciences, analyzed by the 2015 Nobel laureate in economics, Angus Deaton, showing that the death rate among middle-aged, middle-class white people has increased by 22 percent in just the past fifteen years.[1] The leading cause of death in this population is overdose of narcotic drugs and alcohol, whether intentional or accidental. No group of people anywhere in the world in our modern era has shown an increase in the death rate to this extent, and no population in history has shown such a great increase in the death rate in such a short time, with the exception of a disease epidemic or an ecological calamity of global proportions.

In addition, popular over-the-counter pain relievers like acetaminophen (Tylenol, Panadol) have long been known to be the leading cause of fatal liver toxicity in the United States; even worse is recent research showing that these medications are not even effective for back pain and other common pain conditions.

WHAT IS PAIN?

Pain is a complex perceptual phenomenon and the dynamic product of multiple neural circuits, as pain signals are transmitted in specialized nerve receptors along neurons, modulated at all levels of the nervous system, and finally processed in the higher cortical brain centers. Until very recently doctors and researchers said they could not locate any specific "pain center" in the brain. However, in 2015, scientists at the University of Oxford, England, identified an area of pain or a pain center in the brain located in the dorsal (top portion of the brain) posterior insular cortex. Activity in this area of the brain matched study participants' self-reported pain-rating intensities. Researchers were able to find this area by developing a new method of tracking brain activity, which allowed more complex brain states to be analyzed. The results show that it may be possible to help control pain perception directly in the brain.[2]

Acute pain is the result of active tissue damage and the release of inflammatory and chemical pain mediators in any pain-sensitive tissue. Chronic pain states may result from a number of different processes occurring in the peripheral and central nervous-system tissues. Chronic pain may result from an abnormal peripheral or central pain "generator." This type of pain is generally called "neuropathic pain."

THE PERSONALITY BOUNDARY TYPE

Fortunately, there are safe, natural, affordable alternatives for relieving pain that are readily available today and have been hiding in plain sight. To learn which mind-body natural approaches will work best for you, it is important to understand a psychometric indicator developed over several decades at Tufts University Medical Center in Boston by the late Ernest Hartmann, MD, called "personality boundary type." The application of this concept is related to the hypnotic susceptibility or suggestibility scales developed in the last century by American psychiatrist Herbert Spiegel, which have proven useful in predicting which 10 percent of patients are highly benefited by hypnosis, which 10 percent are impervious, and which 80 percent fall on a scale in between. Marc Micozzi and colleague Michael Jawer coined the term *emotional type* for the Hartmann boundary-type psychometric scale and adapted it to predict each person's susceptibility to various kinds of alternative, nondrug treatments. The interactive tools that allow you to determine your individual boundary or emotional psychometric type, together with an assessment for matching your type to the most effective treatments currently available, are provided in this first chapter.

Two essential truths you should know as you embark on this book are the following: (1) most chronic pain results from both the reception of pain signals by pain sensors in the body and the perception and processing of pain sensation in the mind through nerve circuits in the brain and through various levels of consciousness; and (2) the reception and the perception of pain occur in a feedback loop, each continually aggravating the other until chronic pain is permanently cemented in place. The many mind-body therapies presented in this book can each work for most chronic pain conditions because they address these vital linkages, and the feedback loops between the mind and the body. However, not every mind-body therapy works equally well for everyone with chronic pain.

This brings us to the real breakthrough of finding an effective method of choosing from among all these safe and effective therapies the specific ones that will work best for you as a unique individual, and for your pain condition.

We have just now discovered an important way of understanding how the mind-body perceives and processes pain, as well as emotions, moods, and other feelings that affect and reflect our health. Ernest Hartmann worked over his long career on identifying and understanding the psychological and personality boundaries that affect how we process our feelings, emotions, and sensations. He found that people's boundaries exist along a continuum of thin boundary to thick boundary on a spectrum of feelings and experiences—that is, how feelings are experienced and how experiences are felt. For example, Hartmann found that thin boundary people tend to be more artistic, more connected to their dreams, and more likely to see themselves "merge" in their relationships with others. Thick boundary people see clear divides between themselves and others and tend to see the world in black and white. People with thin boundaries are more susceptible to dozens of illnesses with stronger mind-body components, such as irritable bowel syndrome.

For the past twenty years Jawer has researched how it is that people with different boundary types are susceptible to different diseases and chronic pain conditions. Micozzi's own review of thousands of research studies on natural therapies for six editions of his medical textbook *Fundamentals of Complementary and Alternative Medicine,* together with his understanding of the Hartmann-Jawer boundary types, has enabled the authors of this book to now determine which therapies will work best for you based on where you lie on this mind-body boundary-type spectrum. However, please note that the studies cited on the techniques addressed in this book have not distinguished thick from thin boundary types. Everyone gets thrown together in these studies regardless of boundary type. The fact that they work for people of all types is a powerful indicator of their benefits. We would only expect that study results would be even stronger when study participants are matched to the right therapy for each person.

A LITTLE BACKGROUND ON BOUNDARY TYPES

Boundaries are critical because, simply put, our "selves" require boundaries. Just as the skin is a boundary that protects our body from the outside environment, we also need boundaries around our heart energy and our mental consciousness, particularly when it comes to pain. Your sensitivities and reactions to external stimuli and internal states, especially pain, are determined by your qualities as a thin or thick emotional type. Thin boundary people are highly sensitive in a variety of ways and from an early age. Thick boundary people, on the other hand, are typically described as implacable, rigid, stolid, and thick-skinned. That does not mean that thick boundary people do not feel emotions. They may be unaware of them—but their bodies know. For each healing modality we discuss, we will describe why it would be suitable for certain boundary types (and perhaps not for others) and why it works for those types.

THE BOUNDARY QUESTIONNAIRE

As mentioned, the original BQ was developed by Ernest Hartmann based on research he conducted in the 1980s. The full version consists of 145 questions grouped into a dozen categories, reflecting themes such as "interpersonal," "thoughts/feelings/moods," "childhood/adolescence/ adult," and "sleep/dream/waking" (see appendix A on page 227 for the full questionnaire). So, one can be a thin or thick boundary person overall but score differently along the boundary spectrum within these different categories. No one is reducible to a single "spot" on the boundary spectrum. Each of us is likely to be thin in some respects and thick in others.[3]

Where you place on the boundary spectrum is not strictly speaking a permanent position over your lifetime. People tend to develop thicker boundaries as they age, but everyone is different. A person may instead develop thinner boundaries as she gets older based on her unique experiences. Someone's boundaries can even thicken or become thinned based on the medications she takes, or depending on how tired she happens to be.[4] However, as a general personality trait, your boundary type won't vary too much from day to day or from year to year.

A short form of the BQ is presented here. It consists of eighteen questions and usually takes under ten minutes to complete and score. For a quick way to assess your boundary type, the short-form BQ is easiest and most direct.[5] We have found that this subset of eighteen questions captures most of the spectrum variability that is obtained in taking the complete, lengthy survey—that is, each of these particular questions in the short survey is highly correlated to the results of the total answers on the other 127 possible questions that are in the long survey. Moreover, the precision of this short survey is comparable to the precision of the research studies that assessed the effectiveness of different mind-body therapies for different pain conditions, which we used in evaluating their association with a specific boundary type.

Please note that there are no "right" or "wrong" responses. Consider these statements merely as prompts intended to feel you out as to where you are at this time in your life. Rate each of the statements from 0 to 4 (0 indicates "not at all true of me"; 4 indicates "very true of me").

Try to respond to all of the statements as quickly as you can.

SHORT-FORM BOUNDARY QUESTIONNAIRE

1. My feelings blend into one another.   0 1 2 3 4

2. I am very close to my childhood feelings.   0 1 2 3 4

3. I am easily hurt.   0 1 2 3 4

4. I spend a lot of time daydreaming, fantasizing, or in reverie.   0 1 2 3 4

5. I like stories that have a definite beginning, middle, and end.   0 1 2 3 4

6. A good organization is one in which all the lines of responsibility are precise and clearly established.   0 1 2 3 4

7. There should be a place for everything, with everything in its place.   0 1 2 3 4

8. Sometimes it's scary to get too involved with another person.   0 1 2 3 4

9. A good parent has to be a bit of a child too.   0 1 2 3 4

10. I can easily imagine myself as an animal or what it might be like to be an animal.   0 1 2 3 4

11. When something happens to a friend of mine or to a lover, it is almost as if it happened to me.   0 1 2 3 4

12. When I work on a project, I don't like to tie myself down to a definite outline. I rather like to let my mind wander.   0 1 2 3 4

13. In my dreams, people sometimes merge into each other or become other people.   0 1 2 3 4

14. I believe I am influenced by forces that no one can
    understand.   0 1 2 3 4

15. There are no sharp dividing lines between normal people,
    people with problems, and people who are considered   0 1 2 3 4
    psychotic or crazy.

16. I am a down-to-earth, no-nonsense kind of person.   0 1 2 3 4

17. I think I would enjoy being some kind of creative artist.   0 1 2 3 4

18. I have had the experience of someone calling me or
    speaking my name and not being sure whether it was   0 1 2 3 4
    really happening or whether I was imagining it.

To obtain your score, simply add up the scores from 0 to 4 for all questions. **The exceptions are questions 5, 6, 7, and 16, which are scored backward; i.e., for these questions the rating is reversed, such that a score of 0 is scored as 4, a 1 is a 3, a 2 is (still) a 2, a 3 is a 1, and a 4 is scored as 0.** Scores below 30 are considered definitely indicative of a thick boundary, and scores above 42 are considered definitely thin. Find out where you are on the spectrum below:

THICK BOUNDARY----------------------MIDDLE------------------------THIN BOUNDARY

0   9   18   27   36   45   54   63   72

It turns out that your boundary type is related to the effectiveness of each of the common mind-body treatments for pain disorders based on our review of available research and scientific evidence. As you will learn from reading this book, there are many alternative mind-body medical treatments being studied for pain. Each of the treatments presented here is well established, safe, and effective and is rapidly becoming widely available. The effectiveness of each of these treatments for pain is evaluated on the basis of what has by now been

---

*To have your scores automatically calculated, go to www.drmicozzi.com and take the quick Your Emotional Type survey.

proven. This information is provided as a useful guide for you. We do not get into any experimental or controversial treatments here. We are addressing only *proven* treatments that are widely available and have been used for decades, if not longer. The added benefit is that now you can determine which of these treatments is right for you based on your boundary type. If you find a treatment on this list, it is a reasonable that you can safely try it out.

THE RIGHT TREATMENTS FOR YOUR TYPE

Listed here in terms of their effectiveness are some of the major mind-body treatments for common and significant pain disorders. Then we score the degree of specificity for each treatment for your boundary type. Armed with this guide and knowledge of your boundary type, you can begin to select the right treatments for your specific pain condition.

The tables on page 18 show thick and thin boundary conditions, as well as the anxiety and depression that usually accompany all these disorders, and the relative effectiveness of each therapeutic modality for each of these conditions. Based on the available science and research, the treatments are ranked by their effectiveness and potencies on a scale of 1 to 5 relative to one another and relative to the most powerful treatments conventional medicine has to offer in terms of drugs, various procedures, and surgery (even when drugs and surgery are successful, which oftentimes they are not—and they are far more dangerous than any of these treatments). A 1 represents treatments that are somewhat effctive; a 5 represents those that are highly effective. Where no number appears it generally means there is not enough data to evaluate it.

The symptom of chronic pain, as shown in the boundary-independent conditions, typically accompanies all of the specific disorders, and virtually all of these therapies are highly potent and effective for pain. The degree to which they can help you as an individual should be matched to your specific condition and emotional type, since a key to managing pain is treating the underlying condition. In fact, in our view these treatments equal—and acupuncture (for one) actually exceeds—anything available in regular medical treatment for pain. They are highly effective and extremely safe and interfere only minimally with life compared to other pain-management treatments. Furthermore, unlike effective drugs taken for pain, they are not regulated by intrusive government agencies that routinely place real or manufactured law-enforcement concerns above medical judgment and ethics regarding effective pain management for suffering patients.

THICK BOUNDARY CONDITIONS

Disorder	Hypnosis	Acupuncture	Biofeedback	Meditation/ Yoga	Guided Imagery	Relaxation/ Stress Reduction
Rheumatoid Arthritis		3	3	4		3
CFS		3	3	3	3	
Hypertension	2	1	4	5	2	4
Phantom Pain	1	4	2	2		
Psoriasis	2	3				
Ulcer						3

THIN BOUNDARY CONDITIONS

Disorder	Hypnosis	Acupuncture	Biofeedback	Meditation/ Yoga	Guided Imagery	Relaxation/ Stress Reduction
Asthma/ Allergies	4	5	4	2		
Eczema	4					
Fibromyalgia		3				3
IBS	4	4	3			
Migraine	3	4	5	3	3	2
PTSD	2	3	2	3		3

BOUNDARY-INDEPENDENT CONDITIONS

Disorder	Hypnosis	Acupuncture	Biofeedback	Meditation/ Yoga	Guided Imagery	Relaxation/ Stress Reduction
Depression/ Anxiety	4	3	5	5	3	3
Chronic Pain	5	4	5	4	2	3

Some of these conditions are difficult to manage by any means, such as chronic fatigue syndrome (CFS) and fibromyalgia, and the effectiveness and potencies of these active treatments do not reach the highest levels of 4 or 5, although they are usually still quite helpful. Conventional medicine hasn't had much to offer for decades for either of these conditions, with most doctors having told millions of sufferers that it's "all in their heads." Now that drug companies have developed drugs that purportedly treat these disorders, suddenly these conditions actually do exist to the world of modern mainstream medicine—if they are no longer in the heads of these patients, then they are certainly in their wallets.

For many conditions there is a choice of effective CAM treatments. It is noteworthy that several of the therapies are useful for treating both thick and thin boundary types, as well as the common associated conditions of anxiety and depression. However, hypnosis generally does better for treating thin boundary conditions, while it appears that guided imagery, meditation and yoga, and relaxation and stress management generally do better with thick boundary conditions. Biofeedback appears equally effective with both, and acupuncture appears to be a powerhouse across the board for these conditions, although it is even more effective for thin boundary types.

A "Point" about Acupuncture

An important reason why acupuncture does not always work for everyone is because modern cookbook recipes for the way acupuncture is frequently practiced by Westerners do not capture the full scope of available approaches and potencies available in the full spectrum of traditional Chinese medicine (TCM). While it is true that individuals vary in their sensitivities to acupuncture by thick or thin boundary type, among other characteristics—this approach to boundary types sheds new light on this two-thousand-year-old, effective medical tradition—there's more to it than that.

When in research or practice we have observed that "acupuncture just doesn't work" or that it "doesn't work for this person," we simply have taken it at face value in light of general acceptance that CAM is not as "potent" as Western biomedicine. However, it also the case that many writers and practitioners of acupuncture in the West have taken an incomplete approach to the ancient Chinese sources of this time-honored medical tradition. Much of acupuncture practice in the West is incomplete or incorrect because it has been based on particular interpretations that often account for only part of the rich body of knowledge available from the ancient Chinese classics on the subject. The result is a somewhat watered-down Western version that is less potent, or less broad, in its applications to different individuals and their pain conditions. When therapeutic problems are encountered with a particular condition or in a particular individual, too often there is an inability to pursue the next steps by consulting the solutions that are available but have remained hidden in the original Chinese medical writings.

When your regular doctor tries a treatment that does not work, does she or he send you away? No—she or he keeps trying. The same should be true in cases of a lack of initial response in Chinese medicine, if we truly know what else to try, rather than relying only on standard recipes with incomplete knowledge or understanding.

It is also remarkable to note, in addition to the improved therapeutic options provided by a full and complete reading of the authentic Chinese sources, the remarkable depth of diagnostic information available. While the Chinese diagnostics are literally foreign to us, they provide a rich, internally consistent, complete description of people's complaints and experiences that has not been reduced to a series of numbers from standardized biomedical tests performed on only a subset of relevant information. Likewise, understanding of these mind-body boundary types helps complete the picture for our understanding of pain and the modern pain disorders addressed in this book.

SPECTRUM OF TREATMENTS ALONG BOUNDARY LINES

THIN------------------MIDPOINT------------------THICK

HYPNOSIS	ACUPUNCTURE	BIOFEEDBACK	GUIDED IMAGERY	RELAXATION/ STRESS REDUCTION	MEDITATION/ YOGA

The preceding graphic shows the treatments that are specific to thin boundary conditions on the left and those specific to thick boundary conditions on the right, with those in between arranged according to their degree of specificity for one or the other. In terms of general treatments for your boundary type, the most strongly specific treatments for thick personality boundaries (in this order) are meditation and yoga, relaxation and stress reduction, and guided imagery. For thin boundary types, hypnosis is the effective therapy of choice for your condition, followed by acupuncture. Biofeedback is equally specific for thick or thin boundaries. You will learn about all these approaches in this book.

YOUR TREATMENT PROFILE

It is notable that the origins of many chronic pain disorders have remained a mystery to mainstream medical science, and effective treatments have remained equally elusive. It is well established in medicine that sometimes it is ultimately the "treatment profile" of a disease that ultimately provides clues to help backtrack to its etiology, or origins (a process known as "reverse analysis"). That is, once effective treatments are found clinically, they often lead to a better understanding of the causes of the disease. Said differently, once we figure out how to cure the disease, it gives clues as to what is really causing it in the first place.

Now that we can apply the thin and thick boundary concepts to disorders and their treatments, we have another window into what causes these disorders in the first place.

Hypnosis: A 250-Year-Old Mystery Explained

Hypnosis provides a good example of what is conveyed in this book. As with the other mind-body therapies, its mechanism of action has not been known or understood. Again, there is a good reason why this important, effective therapy has had an unknown mechanism of action: the view of neuroscience regarding the brain, mind, and body remains incomplete. Neuroscience has been disregarding critical scientific observations, clinical experiences, and everyday awareness, all of which are central to how our mind-body truly functions.

First developed in the late eighteenth century by German physician Franz Anton Mesmer in Vienna and brought to Paris, to the court of Louis XVI, the use of "animal magnetism" to help people with mind-body disorders proved compelling. However, the "mesmerism," "animal magnetism," and "magnetic healing" of the nineteenth century were all consigned to the dustbin of history by the self-proclaimed "scientific" medical establishment of the twentieth century. Nonetheless, that the potency of hypnotism for problems for which drugs or psychosurgery (such as the notorious frontal lobotomies of the mid-twentieth century) had no answers led serious contemporary psychiatrists and psychologists to again develop and use hypnotism to help their patients.

In the absence of a complete understanding of how hypnotism and mind-body medicine really work, the doctors Herbert Spiegel and his son, David Spiegel, at Stanford University in Palo Alto, California, developed "hypnotic susceptibility scales" to help practitioners predict who and what types of disorders would benefit from this treatment. This breakthrough provided the comfort of proving statistical associations where a more fundamental, mechanistic medical science was lacking.

After nearly a quarter of a century we have now discovered that the susceptibility of individuals to hypnosis relates to boundary type—again, based on statistical associations. Furthermore, you can now apply your understanding of your boundary type to the other common and effective mind-body treatments considered in this book. And you can use these discoveries to seek better, more effective treatments that are tailored to you.

YOUR GUIDE TO MANAGING YOUR PAIN

This chapter provides you with a clear guide as to which type of treatment you probably want to use depending on your boundary type and your medical condition(s).

If you are a thin boundary personality you probably want to try hypnosis or acupuncture first for fibromyalgia or migraine headache, knowing that there are other treatments to try for almost all of these conditions if need be. We have also found that, like the personality/ emotional-type boundaries themselves, fibromyalgia and CFS exist along a spectrum. We have discovered that if you are thick boundary type, you are more likely to experience symptoms toward the CFS end of the spectrum. If you are a thin boundary type, you are likely to experience the syndrome on the fibromyalgia end of the spectrum.

Seen also as spiritual problems in the context of this book, it is clear that both anxiety and depression are amenable to every modality of treatment offered in this book.

All things being equal, start with the highest numbers (for effectiveness), see which treatments work for your condition, start with the effective treatment that best matches your boundary type, and then go on from there as needed.

Now you can see that, as with other things in life, really knowing your boundaries is an important key to health, healing, and happiness.

2
Relaxation and Stress Reduction

The term *stress* was brought into the popular lexicon as a result of the pioneering work of Austrian-Canadian endocrinologist Hans Selye (1907–1982), who served as director of the Institute of Experimental Medicine and Surgery at the University of Montreal. Selye adapted the term from mechanical engineering and applied it to human health to refer to "the rate of wear and tear on the body."[1] The debate continues as to whether stress is what causes the wear and tear, or whether it is the result of it. Selye explained the stress response in terms of what he called the "general adaption syndrome," or GAS, which describes a way of adapting or adjusting to changes in the environment. GAS has three phases: an alarm reaction, a stage of resistance, and a stage of exhaustion. A stress cause, or stressor, mobilizes GAS by activating the sympathetic part of the autonomic nervous system, thereby releasing adrenaline (epinephrine) hormones. These hormones bring about physiological changes in the body, which Selye described as the "fight-or-flight response."[2] As a result, the emotional state of stress may actually become embodied throughout one's being.[3]

The problem of stress has continued to draw attention from the media over the years. We have also heard the cliché that stress was the epidemic of the 1980s and 1990s. Back in 1970, American writer and futurist Alvin Toffler, in his book *Future Shock,* posited that humans had already reached their maximum capacity to tolerate change and stress. In that case we may need an entirely new term to describe the experience of the twenty-first century thus far!

Over the years it has become apparent that stress is the cause of chronic conditions such as cardiovascular disease, diabetes, and many forms of cancer. But the academic-government-industrial-medical complex continues to spread the myth that cholesterol, fats, and salt are the primary causes of chronic disease, even though there has never been any real evidence to support these claims. Meanwhile, *stress* has become a buzzword. All the alarmist and negative publicity has stimulated further anxiety and concern in many people's minds—a fear of stress itself, which leads to even more stress. Having been made aware of the problem, everyone now wants to manage stress, and many (perhaps too many) cater to this growing market. This rapidly growing segment includes various self-styled experts, management consultants, New Age gurus, Johnny-come-lately physicians, and others. Vitamin regimens, herbal supplements, energy beverages, fitness programs, relaxation techniques, life coaching, and personal development courses are all being offered in the quest for stress control. All sorts of experts are convinced that their particular product or service can banish stress for good. In the land of the blind, the one-eyed man is king. Part of the problem is that the so-called experts have been working without a complete understanding of what we see as the "spiritual anatomy" of emotions that lie at the heart of the experience of stress.[4]

The fact remains that there are no magic cures and no silver bullets. Stress is essentially a result of an interaction between a negative environment, an unhealthful lifestyle, and self-defeating attitudes and beliefs. Therefore, unlike what is believed by stress management consultants and other experts, no one particular technique, method, program, or regimen can eliminate long-term stress.

A growing trend, in part due to its simplicity and its effectiveness, is mindfulness-based meditation and mindfulness-based stress reduction (MBSR), part of the rapidly growing field of mindfulness-based interventions (MBIs).[5] Throughout the world there are now different practices that bring wonderful new insights into how anyone can live with whatever stress is in their life. These different approaches to mindfulness are the single most effective and accessible methods for dealing with stress, and they can be practiced anytime, anywhere.[6]

WHAT IS STRESS?

Stress is most often seen as the end result of outside pressures and problems that encroach on our busy lives: deadlines, excessive work, noise, traffic, pollution, problems with family or friends, and excessive demands made by others. Stress involves the unconscious response to these kinds of pressures. Ultimately, stress is not "those things out there," but rather what happens inside our minds and bodies as we react unconsciously to those situations that we experience as stressful.

Normally we experience some degree of stress in everything we do and everything that happens to us. Research shows that within reasonable limits, some stress ("eustress," or positive stress) is helpful in bringing about adaptive changes in the way our minds and bodies work. In *Magical Child,* published in 1977, American author Joseph Chilton Pearce wrote that "stress is the way intelligence grows."[7] He explains that under stress the brain immediately grows massive numbers of new connecting links between the neurons that enable learning. Although the stressed mind/brain grows in ability and the unstressed mind lags behind, the overstressed mind/brain can collapse into physiological shock. Essential to this delicate balance in maintaining an optimal level of stress is relaxation.

When the stress response is minor, we do not notice any symptoms. The greater the stimulation, the more symptoms we notice. In the 1960s, psychiatrists Thomas Holmes and Richard Rahe's scale of life changes, published as the Social Readjustment Rating Scale, provided a guide to the amount of stress attached to major life events such as marriage, relocation, emigration, loss of a job, death of a spouse, or birth of a child. These significant life events, whether we judge them as positive, negative, or neutral, can quickly overload our ability to cope.

In *The Human Zoo,* English zoologist and ethologist Desmond Morris wrote that modern humans are engaged in what he called the "stimulus struggle": "If we abandon it [the struggle], or tackle it badly, we are in serious trouble."[8] We are trying to maintain the optimal level of stimulation—not the maximum, but the right level, one that is most beneficial, somewhere between understimulation and overstimulation.

Stress becomes a problem when it reaches excessive levels, when the demands exceed our ability to respond or to cope effectively. When we are under excessive, prolonged stress and no longer are able to cope or adjust, stress becomes distress. Imbalances then develop that lead to stress-induced symptoms, illnesses, and diseases. The physical body's engine begins to rev at high speed, totally absorbing restricted, unproductive energy. Over extended periods, this wear and tear begins to take its toll, opening the way for diseases to creep into the body.

Change and Stress

We can learn to control our response to stress by changing the way we think. Stress management includes developing the ability to assert control over our behavior. When we become aware of our ability to control attitudes and behaviors, we naturally begin to assert control over life situations that once seemed stressful. It is not the stress itself that is harmful, but our reaction to it that wreaks havoc in the body, mind, and spirit.

The greatest stressor that most people experience daily is change, yet the only thing constant in life is change. Frustration and feelings of loss, grief, and suffering are among the many unconscious responses to change. Change is inevitable and continually requires you to adapt to new situations. If you do not adapt to change by altering your attitude, then both mind and body suffer. When change takes place in your environment, career, and personal relationships, it becomes essential to learn how to behave, think, and feel differently to cope with the new situation effectively.

We are each continuously adjusting to changing conditions, rather like a thermostat. As the weather outside changes, the thermostat turns the heater or air conditioner on, down, or up, which brings the interior temperature back to a specified level of comfort. The greater the change outside, the harder the furnace or air conditioner has to work to keep up with it. If the external temperature moves into an extreme range, the system will be pushed to the max. If it exceeds its specified limit, it will eventually break down and burn out. So it is with the human body. Your body continuously reacts to whatever is happening around you or inside you. You respond physically, mentally, and emotionally to even the most minute changes. This process occurs all the time, whether you are consciously aware of it or not.

Stress is a very subjective condition. No two people respond to life's ups and downs in the same way. We know people who can remain cool, calm, and collected under the most trying circumstances, and we know others who are unable to cope when faced with even minor situations. The differences may result from different upbringings, past understandings, present experiences, attitudes, belief structures, family values, perceptions, coping skills developed over years and generations, and the simple matter of aging. For example, spending money shopping is extremely stressful for some people, while for others it's a joyful experience and a way of actually adapting or responding to stress.

Furthermore, some people have a higher stress tolerance than others. We know that type A personalities are naturally high-strung and react strongly to stress, and that type B personalities are more easygoing and can better tolerate stress. Back in the 1950s, researchers found that these two basic behavior patterns affect health. In fact, they found that type A personalities are more likely to develop coronary heart disease than type Bs.

We also now recognize there are type C personalities. These are people who actually deny their feelings of stress. Outwardly, they appear cool, relaxed, and totally in control of their surroundings and themselves. But by ignoring their stress, they wind up heightening their risk of developing all the major health problems mentioned above. (Of course, there is one other "type"—the type who says, "I don't get heart attacks, I give them.") All this can make stress hard to pin down. We believe that the psychometric personality boundary type developed by psychoanalyst Ernest Hartmann, as described in chapter 1, along with our simple psychometric profile questionnaire, will be the single best way for you to find out which specific disorders stress may cause in you, thereby indicating which mind-body therapies will work best for you in managing these stress-related disorders. We also use another tool to measure stress, called the "life change index scale," from Holmes and Rahe, which can easily be found online. This tool counts and scores major life changes that occur during the course of a lifetime. A higher score—meaning more major life changes—means you run a greater risk of heart attack and various diseases during the period in which these stresses occur.

Interestingly, this index measures major life changes, both good and bad, not just negative life changes. That's because the body experiences stress as stress. It doesn't distinguish between a wedding and a divorce, or between a new job versus a layoff. We might interpret a given change as "good" or "bad," but our body does not make this distinction.

We also use another tool for diagnosing stress: our own feelings. It turns out that some people can be very good at judging whether they feel stressed. In fact, in a recent study conducted in the United Kingdom, researchers asked men and women if they experienced high stress. If the subjects said "yes," the researchers discovered that this response accurately predicted future heart problems.[9] Sometimes, when doctors or scientists struggle to understand stress in people, they might just try asking them!

Overall, humans are largely creatures of habit. We do not respond well to change, positive or negative. And even the most unique characters among us are somewhat wired for conformity. For example, when you see someone laugh or smile, most of us tend to return the smile. Or when your partner—or even your pet—yawns, chances are you will too. So naturally when you work with stressed-out colleagues, you feel stressed out, too.

Your Brain on Stress

The interconnectedness you see among humans is unique to large animals who live at the top of the food chain (this group includes canines). We work in groups rather than alone. And as social animals, our brains are biologically wired to relate to others, whether laughing, yawning, or panicking. This is because our brains have what are known as "mirror neurons." These highly evolved brain cells react by mimicking the actions and emotions of others. Thus the neurons "mirror" the behavior of the others, as though the observer were itself acting.

Italian scientists first identified mirror neurons in the 1980s and 1990s. From studying macaque monkeys they learned that specific groups of neurons in the brain (mirror neurons) lit up when the monkeys performed, or even just observed, specific types of movements. It turns out that mirror neurons in monkeys as well as humans are located near motor neurons. So, reflected behaviors directly affect our movements, our speech, and even our emotions—giving new meaning to the old adage "monkey see, monkey do."

This kind of mirror reflection is one reason why stress is highly contagious. Researchers have observed the almost infectious nature of stress for a long time, but now we know something about how and why it happens. Anxiety appears to spread like a virus. Crossover stress occurs between spouses and among co-workers. Stress can also spill over from the workplace to the home, and vice versa.

We process stress in a core of the ancient, "reptilian" brain that we can't consciously control. It simply cannot rationalize the stresses of the modern world. No wonder stress factors into five out of six of the leading causes of death. Even government agencies like the U.S. Centers for Disease Control and Prevention now recognize that stress kills more people than traffic accidents or smoking—despite the fact that the government is increasingly obsessed with antitobacco campaigns while virtually ignoring the stress that is killing us (and meanwhile the government itself is an increasing source of stress for most Americans).

When someone dumps their emotional stress onto you, instead of latching on to it, take a step back and reframe the story to reality. Someone else's irrational stress is not your emergency. Use your more evolved rational brain instead of allowing your reptilian brain to call the shots. This approach can be equated to using logic over emotion. Logic is associated with the prefrontal cortex, where executive functions like planning and decision making also take place, whereas emotional responses are found in the amygdala, or reptilian brain, which is associated with the processing of fear, negative emotions, emotional behaviors, and emotional responses.

The Symptoms of Stress

When someone experiences distress, the symptoms are unique to that person. Different people appear to channel excessive stress into different parts of the body. The long-term effects of these different responses include various physical illnesses, including chronic backache, headache, high blood pressure, ulcers, or other chronic disorders. Decades of research have linked stress, either directly or indirectly, to coronary heart disease, cancer, stroke, lung ailments, injuries from accidents, cirrhosis of the liver, immune-system deficiencies, and suicide. Whether it is either a precursor of disease or an outcome of it, stress is often a component of chronic illness. People who can manage stress are more physically resilient, have fewer symptoms, and experience an improved quality of life.

Testing the effects of meditation on hypertension, researchers have found that all meditation techniques are equally effective in treating high blood pressure or hypertension. But when prescribed in the absence of further nondrug interventions, meditation techniques were not as effective as standard antihypertensive drug pharmacotherapy. The key, of course, is matching the specific techniques to your individual personality boundary type, or emotional type.[10] They all have the potential to work when properly matched to the boundary type, while none may work well—or even work at all—if incorrectly matched to the person.

Herbert Benson, founder of the Mind/Body Medical Institute at Massachusetts General Hospital in Boston and professor of mind/body medicine at Harvard Medical School, first began investigating the benefits of stress reduction and relaxation in the late 1960s, and he continues to delve into the effects of stress on various disease-specific populations. Benson's group has specifically examined the stress phenomenon and its effect on cardiovascular and neurodegenerative diseases.[11] They found that stress has a major impact on the circulatory and nervous systems, playing a significant role in the susceptibility to and progress and outcome of both cardiovascular and neurodegenerative diseases. However, they also found that some amounts of stress (eustress) can actually improve performance and thus can be beneficial in certain cases.

A 2013 study out of Sweden adds another illness to the list—and it's not one you might normally associate with stress. Researchers in Sweden, which has good health care and high-quality medical research, did a study on how stress affects women's health. The study considered factors like divorce, life stress, and health issues involving family matters. The researchers studied eight hundred middle-aged women—a good size for a longitudinal sample (repeated observations of the same variables over long periods of time, often many decades, in the same sample of people)—over a period of four decades. They found that the effects of stressful events are not short-lived. In fact, stress in middle age makes a person more susceptible to developing Alzheimer's disease decades later. How this connection may work is that through its effects on certain hormones, chronic stress can change the workings of the brain circuitry. This effect, in turn, may leave people more susceptible to the impact of Alzheimer's-type brain changes at older ages.[12]

According to the American Institute of Stress, during the past decade, workplace stress has led to $300 billion a year in health care costs as a result of missed work alone. During the same time period the National Institute for Occupational Safety and Health (part of the Department of Health and Human Services of the Centers for Disease Control and Prevention) claimed that stressed workers incurred health care costs nearly 50 percent higher than nonstressed employees, an average of $600 more per person.

THE CURE FOR STRESS: THE RELAXATION RESPONSE

Believing that benefits of meditation and relaxation could potentially lower high blood pressure, Herbert Benson researched a variety of psychological and physiological effects that appear common to many mind-body practices. In the 1970s he coined the term *relaxation response* (and wrote a 1975 book by the same title), a scientific term that describes the ability of the body to stimulate relaxation of muscles and organs, a response common to different forms of meditation, prayer, autogenic training, and some forms of hypnosis. Benson's research indicated that excessive stress could cause or aggravate hypertension and its related diseases—atherosclerosis, heart attack, and stroke. He then examined the nature of the relaxation response, showing that the physiological changes that take place during true relaxation include the lowering of the rates of oxygen consumption, metabolism, heartbeat, and blood pressure, as well as increased production of alpha brain waves. A marked decrease in blood lactate (lactic acid) was also found; notably, high blood lactate has often been linked to anxiety.

Benson suggests the follow technique to elicit the relaxation response.

❀ Generating the Relaxation Response

Try to find ten to twenty minutes in your daily routine to do this exercise; before breakfast is generally a good time.

For the period you will practice, try to arrange your life so that you will have no distractions. For example, let the answering machine handle the phone, turn your phone to silent or airplane mode, or ask someone to watch the children.

Time yourself by glancing periodically at a clock or watch (but do not set an alarm). Commit yourself to a specific length of practice.

Step 1: Sit quietly in a comfortable position.

Step 2: Pick a focus word or short phrase that is firmly rooted in your personal belief system. For example, a nonreligious person might choose a neutral word such as *oneness, peace,* or *love.* A Christian wanting to use a prayer could pick the opening words of Psalm 23, "The Lord is my shepherd"; a Jewish person might choose the word *shalom* ("peace").

Step 3: Close your eyes.

Step 4: Relax your muscles.

Step 5: Breathe slowly, deeply, and naturally, repeating your focus word or phrase silently every time you exhale.

Step 6: Throughout, assume a passive attitude. Do not worry about how well you are doing. When other thoughts come to mind, simply say to yourself, "Oh, well," and gently return to the repetition.

Step 7: Continue in this way for ten to twenty minutes. You may open your eyes once in a while to check the time, but do not use a timer. When you finish, sit quietly for a minute or so, at first with your eyes closed and later with your eyes open. Do not stand up for at least one or two minutes.

Step 8: Practice this technique once or twice a day.

Benson's research into the relaxation response has covered several other efficient techniques for relaxation, including Transcendental Meditation (TM), Zen, yoga, progressive relaxation, hypnosis, and others as illustrated in the table below. He found that each of these methods had four elements in common: a quiet environment, an object on which to focus the mind, a passive attitude, and a comfortable position.[13] Some practices are more effective than others, partially depending on boundary types, and some are easier to learn and practice than others.

RELAXATION RESPONSE

Technique	Oxygen Consumption	Respiratory Rate	Heart Rate	Alpha Waves	Blood Pressure	Muscle Tension
Transcendental Meditation	decreases	decreases	decreases	increase	decreases*	(not measured)
Zen and yoga	decreases	decreases	decreases	increase	decreases*	(not measured)
autogenic training (biofeedback)	(not measured)	decreases	decreases	increase	inconclusive	(not measured)
progressive relaxation	(not measured)	(not measured)	(not measured)	(not measured)	inconclusive	decreases
hypnosis with deep relaxation	decreases	decreases	decreases	(not measured)	inconclusive	(not measured)

*In patients with elevated blood pressure.

Exercise for Stress Reduction

Michael Sacks, MD, professor of psychiatry at Weill Cornell Medical Center and attending psychiatrist at the New York Presbyterian Hospital, found that various forms of exercise can be powerful methods of relaxation that are effective in dealing with the stress of daily life. Researchers found in various studies that exercise can decrease anxiety and depression, improve a person's self-image, and buffer people from the effects of stress. Taken as a whole, the body of research strongly supports the fact that exercise can elevate mood and reduce anxiety and stress.[14]

Although most research has largely focused on the physical benefits of exercise, exercise can also help people feel more focused and at the same time more relaxed, as long as the activity is enjoyable. And regular exercise does seem to affect one aspect in particular: the ability to withstand stress. Exercise and physical fitness can act as a buffer against stress so that stressful events have a less negative impact on psychological and physical health.

THE PROVEN EFFECTIVENESS
OF STRESS REDUCTION

Benson's group found that patients with chronic pain who meditated regularly had a net reduction in general health care costs, suggesting that the effects of relaxation techniques are cost-effective, but this is only one of the many benefits of these techniques. Drug-resistant epileptic patients who practiced Benson's relaxation response for twenty minutes each day experienced decreased frequency of seizures, increasing significantly with six to twelve months of continued practice. The duration of seizures also declined over twelve months. The value of Benson's technique for patients with heart failure was evidenced in a study in nearly sixty veterans who received relaxation-response training. Approximately half of this group reported physical improvements that went beyond disease management and into lifestyle changes and improved relationships.[15]

Benson and his team of researchers also discovered that relaxation actually causes the genes in our cells to switch into a different mode.[16] In other words, by generating a relaxation response you can actually regulate your genes to kick in to counteract the toxic effects of stress. (This effect, by the way, may explain the long-observed profound control that certain advanced yogis develop over all their vital functions.)

Benson's group of researchers noted four specific types of genetic responses to relaxation. The first involved genes related to mitochondria, which power the cells. This response resulted in better mood, energy, and sleep in the subjects who meditated. The second gene response was seen in genes linked to insulin. This effect boosted energy in the cells by regulating all-important blood-sugar metabolism. So responses one and two together influence the most basic energy processes of the body: oxygenation through cellular respiration in the mitochondria, and carbohydrate metabolism for useful calories. Third, researchers found that people who meditated had less activity in genes that turn on the inflammatory response. In other words, their immune systems were better modulated, or balanced. An imbalanced immune system and chronic inflammation may very well be the primary cause of persistent chronic problems such as heart disease and cancer. And finally, meditation also influenced genes related to telomeres in the cells. Telomeres cap off the ends of chromosomes and protect your cells' genetic material (DNA), especially during cell division and multiplication. Cells are continually dividing and multiplying in order to replace older, worn-out cells with newer, healthy cells. This means they are directly related to longevity. Meditation can therefore extend your life span, as has been observed in yogis and meditators for over a century.

And all it takes is just ten to twenty minutes a day to effect profound benefits.

BOUNDARY TYPES: WHO BENEFITS AND WHY

Certain emotional types may gain greater benefits from relaxation techniques and exercise as described in this chapter. For example, in the table on boundary types in the previous chapter we show that relaxation ("stress reduction") is above the midpoint, closer to thick boundary types. A thick boundary person has to relax to even become aware of what they are feeling. Relaxation-based approaches, it turns out, work better for a number of the thick boundary conditions—because the dissociated feelings underlying them may require relaxation first, in order for the person to be receptive to the possibility that feelings are even at play. A thick boundary often means a person tends to push down his or her feelings such that they go unacknowledged, while a thin type may be hypersensitive to the least little stressor.

FINDING A TEACHER

Relaxation and stress reduction are often taught as a group class over a number of weeks. Generally relaxation and stress reduction are taught by or incorporated into the work of practitioners of other alternative modalities and are not the main modality in and of itself. Relaxation, as you will see in the following chapters, is a necessary precondition for any mind-body therapy work, and most mind-body therapies incorporate elements of relaxation—which contributes to stress reduction.

You can find more on locating practitioners of the correlated mind-body modalities later in this book. You can also search for stress reduction workshops, classes, and groups online using search terms such as "mindfulness-based stress reduction." For more specifics on mindfulness teachers, see "Finding a Teacher" on page 107 in chapter 6.

3
Biofeedback

Biofeedback is a technique and process that enables a person to learn how to change physiological activity for the purposes of improving health and performance. Biofeedback systems have essentially been known in India and other countries for millennia. Ancient Hindu practices like yoga and pranayama (see chapter 6) are basically biofeedback methods. However, biofeedback therapies as we now know them emerged in the 1960s and 1970s, when advances in psychological and medical research converged with developments in biomedical technology. Improved electronic instruments could convey information to patients about their nervous systems and their muscles in the form of audio and visual signals that patients could understand.

The term *biofeedback* was first coined around this same time and came to define the procedures and treatments that make use of these instruments, as articulated in the 1977 book *Beyond Biofeedback*. The very same year that Elmer Green and Alyce Green published this seminal book, I (Micozzi) met them in Laguna de Bay, Luzon, Philippines, at a special World Health Organization conference on Filipino faith healers. I had just traveled to Southeast Asia under a Henry Luce Foundation fellowship when I was literally blown off course in my journey and I ended up at this conference, which was sponsored by the Caliraya Foundation. It was my first introduction to mind-body healing. Also present at the conference was Alan Landsburg, producer of the then new television series *In Search Of,* hosted by the late Leonard Nimoy

(Mr. Spock on *Star Trek*). I realized that not only did the topic of mind-body healing push the boundaries of our concepts of health and healing, it was of great popular interest at the time.

Biofeedback therapy uses special instruments, devices, and methods to expand on the body's natural internal feedback systems. By observing a monitoring device, people can learn by trial and error to adjust their thinking and other mental processes to control bodily processes previously once thought to be entirely involuntary, such as blood pressure, temperature, gastrointestinal functioning, and brain-wave activity.

- Biofeedback can be used on almost any bodily process that can be measured accurately.
- Biofeedback-assisted relaxation training has now been shown to be associated with a decrease in medical-care costs, a decrease in the number of claims and costs to insurers in claims payments, reduction in the use of medications and physician use, reduction in hospital stays and rehospitalizations, reduction of mortality and morbidity, and enhanced quality of life.
- Biofeedback is more useful for some clinical problems than for others, and for some people depending on their mind-body type, as we will review later in this chapter. It has also become an integral part of the treatment of many disorders, including anxiety, asthma, headaches, and muscle pain disorders.
- Biofeedback can be successful in helping people learn to regulate many physical conditions because it puts them in better contact with specific parts of their bodies.

YOU ARE IN CHARGE

The general goal of biofeedback therapy is to lower body tension and change negative biological patterns (which we find are related to emotional-type boundaries, as you will see below) to reduce symptoms. While many people can and do reach goals of relaxation without the use of biofeedback, and biofeedback may not be necessary to accomplish a relaxation response, it can usually add something useful to any treatment.

A major reason why many people find biofeedback training appealing is that, as with behavioral approaches in general, it puts you in the driver's seat, giving you a sense of mastery and self-reliance over any illness. Such an attitude can play a critical role in shortening recovery time, reducing disease incidence, and lowering health care costs for almost any medical condition.

There is strong scientific evidence for the use of biofeedback as a treatment for several chronic pain disorders, particularly tension-type and migraine headaches. The effects of biofeedback may be specific, nonspecific, or both. Nonspecific positive effects include gaining confidence, improved concentration, and more effective coping strategies. The specific effects involve learning to gain control of your individual physiological processes, such as brain waves or muscle tension. In either case the benefit is that you are directly involved in the therapeutic process.

The immediacy and accuracy of the biofeedback information you are provided with is critical, but the relationship between the therapist and the client is equally important in realizing its full potential. People with stress-related pain and mood disorders have acquired maladaptive response patterns that have led to dysfunctional coping and oversensitivity to stress. Especially with thin boundary types suffering from chronic pain, even neutral stimuli may be perceived as threats, so that over time the risk of suffering pain as a result of psychological conflict increases. People who react in maladaptive ways clearly need new coping skills. However, skills may not be enough. Your ability to self-regulate requires more than simply learning a technique; it requires you to make a conceptual shift. You must realize that controlling physiological and psychological responses *is* possible. As you learn to self-regulate, sensory information is processed differently. For example, pain is interpreted directly as a message from the body, not an inevitable prelude to an incapacitating migraine or a global indictment of everything that has ever gone wrong in your life. Your response to the pain message in part involves learning new skills, but it also means making cognitive adjustments that lead to positive psychological responses. Although your practitioner begins with a framework and a standard treatment package in mind, the therapy should be flexible enough to be modified for you as an individual.

HOW IT WORKS

Biofeedback is a mind-body therapy based on classic behavioral-psychology operant learning, in which reflexes are developed to respond to stimuli through the mechanism of feedback, to teach new ways of responding to stress that are helpful and healthy. A biofeedback client receives information about his or her specific physiological function and, with practice, through simple trial and error, learns to control his or her response to stress. Biofeedback requires monitoring and displaying accurate and meaningful information from a body site in an easily read and recognizable form. "Correct" or desired responses and reactions are reinforced by sound or visual feedback, facilitating learning. With the guidance of a biofeedback practitioner and with regular practice, the client can repeatedly and reliably control one or more physiological responses.

For example, muscle tension is measured from the forehead with surface sensors. The output is converted to a visual or auditory signal that is made available to the person, such as a sound that fluctuates depending on the level of tension. Being able to observe and learn which muscles are tense or relaxed allows the person to self-regulate this physiological process. Undesirable internal states are associated with increased levels of sound or light. Reinforcement of desirable internal states is provided for desired responses, such as relaxed muscles.

There are three broad categories of biofeedback treatment: (1) stress reduction, in which lower arousal is reinforced; (2) muscle retraining, in conditions where muscle tone is lower than desired; and (3) brainwave training, for disorders in which EEG patterns are associated with specific problems of attention and concentration.

All biofeedback approaches involve the following:

• A monitoring instrument is utilized.
• The person observes and receives information.

- Correct responses are reinforced (i.e., "operant conditioning").
- Repetition is necessary for optimal results.

Forms of Biofeedback

There are five basic forms of biofeedback therapy:

Electromyographic biofeedback. EMG feedback measures muscular tension. Sensors are attached to the skin to detect electrical activity related to muscle tension in that area. The biofeedback instrument amplifies and converts this activity into useful information, displaying the various degrees of muscle tension in the form of an auditory signal. For disorders in which excessive muscle tension and overarousal are associated with symptoms and lowered responsiveness, surface muscle-tension monitoring by measuring muscular potentials and movements without puncturing the skin is appropriate. However, when the objective is to increase motor muscular activity, needles are often inserted. This form of biofeedback therapy is most often used for tension headaches, physical rehabilitation, chronic pain, incontinence, and general relaxation.

Thermal biofeedback therapy. Thermal biofeedback is used to measure skin temperature as an index of blood flow changes from the constriction and dilation of blood vessels. Low skin temperature usually means decreased blood flow in that area. A temperature-sensitive probe is taped to the skin, often on a finger. The instrument converts information into feedback that can be seen and heard and can be used to reduce or increase blood flow to the hands and feet. Thermal biofeedback is often used for migraine headaches and anxiety disorders and to promote general relaxation.

Electrodermal activity therapy. This is used to measure changes in perspiration activity too minimal to feel. Two sensors are attached to the palm side of the fingers or hand to measure sweat activity. They produce a tiny electrical current that measures skin conductance on the basis of the amount of moisture present. Increased sweat can mean arousal of part of the autonomic nervous system. Electrodermal activity therapy can be used to measure the sweat output stemming from stressful thoughts or rapid deep breathing. It is most often used for anxiety and excessive sweating due to any cause.

Finger pulse therapy. This form of biofeedback measures pulse rate and force. A sensor is attached to a finger to measure heart activity as a sign of arousal of part of the autonomic nervous system. Finger pulse therapy is most often used for anxiety and for some cardiac arrhythmias.

Breathing biofeedback therapy. This measures breath rate, volume, rhythm, and location. Sensors are placed around the chest and abdomen to measure airflow from the mouth and nose. The feedback is usually visual, and the person learns to take deeper, slower, lower, and more regular breaths using abdominal muscles. This simple form of biofeedback is most often used for anxiety.

In addition to these basic forms of biofeedback, brain-wave (electroencephalogram, or EEG) feedback, also called "neurofeedback," involves monitoring brain-wave activity of certain areas of the brain underlying the areas where electrodes are placed.

Heart rate and blood-pressure feedback, as provided, for example, through finger pulse therapy, provides information about the regulation of the cardiovascular system. A newer form of biofeedback is heart-rate variability, which is used to facilitate a person's learning to control the oscillation (variability) of the heart rate. Lower heart rate variability has been linked to cardiovascular disease.

Inducing Relaxation

We all need to be aware of dangers in our environments, including other people, so that we are able to monitor and perceive what we need to react to in order to prevent or avoid adverse outcomes. This is part of using our fight or flight responses. However, long-standing stressors that we perceive as threats can lead to a conservation-withdrawal response often associated with depression and anxiety. When you become hypervigilant, your nervous system is in a "resting" state of overarousal, even when there is no real threat. And this can be hazardous to your health.

When the primary objective is to lower arousal rates, relaxation becomes an integral part of biofeedback therapy. Relaxation that can be achieved by biofeedback is of two basic types: active and passive. Active relaxation is defined as producing lower arousal by voluntarily tensing and releasing tension from specific muscle groups and learning to differentiate between tension and relaxation to consciously lower tension. This approach could also be referred to as "applied relaxation" and "progressive relaxation."

Passive relaxation consists of deep breathing or using words, phrases, or imagery. For example, autogenic relaxation (as in hypnosis) uses specific phrases dealing with sensations of heaviness in the muscles and warmth in the hands, such as "my legs are getting heavier" or "my hands are getting warmer." A key to effective relaxation (as it may also be with meditation) is the repetition of phrases or behavior (such as breathing) on a daily basis until a reliable relaxation response can be produced quickly when needed. Biofeedback responses can also be used to monitor the attainment of passive relaxation, as with breathing patterns.

Home practice of relaxation with or without portable biofeedback devices is critical to learning and long-term maintenance of newly acquired coping skills. Generalization of the relaxation response to conditions of daily living allows a person to use relaxation to counter the effects of stressful situations. The experience of decreasing the severity of a stress response or blocking the response with relaxation rather than relying on medication increases one's confidence in one's own ability to use a given biofeedback technique. Different relaxation techniques have specific effects, and the biofeedback therapist guides the person in learning to differentiate among various responses and to match each signal to a strategy: breathing, passive or active relaxation, or imagery.

What It's Like

In the typical biofeedback training session, electrodes are attached to the area being monitored with the therapist. These electrodes feed the information to a small monitoring box that registers the results by a sound tone that varies in pitch or on a visual meter that varies in brightness as the function being monitored decreases or increases. The biofeedback therapist leads the person in mental exercises to help him or her achieve the desired result. In this way, through trial and error, the person gradually learns how to control the inner mechanism involved in the behavioral response. Training for some disorders requires eight to ten sessions; however, sometimes a single session can provide symptomatic relief. People with long-term or severe pain may require a longer course of therapy. The aim of the treatment is to teach the person to regulate his or her own inner mental and bodily processes, eventually without the help of the biofeedback machine.

Reliable symptom monitoring before, during, and following biofeedback sessions with the therapist is necessary to first establish a baseline, then to monitor the progress of treatment, and finally to determine the outcome. For this reason, in practicing relaxation techniques at home with a biofeedback machine the person records symptoms, and this information is later reviewed with the biofeedback therapist. This kind of symptom monitoring and periodic review with the therapist both informs treatment and serves as a source of reinforcement of the person's progress. A pretreatment baseline can be easily established if the person tracks the frequency, duration, and severity of symptoms and medication use prior to initiating the use of biofeedback. In this way the person becomes fully engaged in the therapeutic process.

The therapist initially provides the person with an explanation of the rationale for biofeedback and how it works. For example, biofeedback for disorders of excessive muscle tension and tension-type headaches is pretty quickly grasped by most people; the relationship between a high-pitched or high-frequency sound and high muscle tension is intuitively obvious. However, other symptom-feedback pairs may be less obvious. For example, a person with a migraine headache who is going to learn to warm her hands with thermal biofeedback might be told something like the following: "When you are in a stressful situation, your body gets ready to react. This reaction includes tensing your muscles, increasing your pulse rate, and sending blood to your muscles. Thus blood is diverted away from internal organs like your digestive system, or your hands and feet. When there is less warm blood in your fingers, they get cold. With feedback, you will learn to warm your hands consciously. This is part of learning how to decrease your response to stress, which seems to be related to your headaches." Warming of a part of the body means there is increased blood flow to that area, typically resulting from relaxation of the blood vessels.

THE PROVEN EFFECTIVENESS OF BIOFEEDBACK THERAPY

Biofeedback is considered a hands-on therapy that facilitates cognitive-behavioral changes that result in relaxation that is of benefit for a wide variety of pain conditions.

Blood Pressure

Blood pressure is related to blood flow, which is related to inflammation and pain. The mind influences blood flow—and therefore blood pressure—by communicating with the small muscles in the arteries and adjusting the blood vessels' tone, size, dimensions, and flow. Biofeedback—along with imagery, relaxation techniques, and meditation—influences blood flow and blood pressure.

Blood flow to the head can be consciously influenced through biofeedback techniques as well as through relaxation. The use of EEG biofeedback for enhanced concentration can also be substantial. This is biofeedback where the data comes from an electroencephalogram, showing brain waves associated with different brain activities and states of consciousness. You can learn to influence your brain-wave activity in a self-directed manner through this method of biofeedback. Its effects have been explained by therapists as, for example, the following: "Certain brain-wave patterns are associated with sleep, others with attention and good concentration, and others with lack of attention or daydreaming. You will be able to learn to generate brain waves that are associated with good concentration and paying attention, instead of being distracted or unfocused."[1]

Depression, Anxiety, Phobias

Depression is characterized by a pervasive and persistent low mood accompanied by low self-esteem and a loss of interest or pleasure in normally enjoyable life activities. It can adversely affect a person's family, work, or school life, sleeping and eating habits, and general health, and it can sometimes lead to suicide. In the United States, it has been found that up to 60 percent of people who die by suicide had depression or some other mood disorder.[2]

Depression is often prominent in people who experience chronic headaches or other pain syndromes. In women, chronic severe headache and resultant disability are associated with depression.[3] A neuro-psycho-chemical association is common to both pain and negative emotional states. Cognitive-behavioral therapy (CBT), a form of talk therapy generally performed in one-on-one sessions with a psychotherapist, is commonly used in conjunction with biofeedback for anxiety and mood disorders. CBT explores negative and irrational thoughts that contribute to mood symptoms and teaches the person to counter these thoughts with more realistic approaches to situations. In so doing this form of therapy emphasizes generating more positive thinking patterns and acquiring effective coping skills.

An intensive biofeedback treatment protocol is often recommended for people who have long-standing moderate or severe symptoms of depression, who are poorly motivated, and whose lives are focused on pain. When pain or disability is severe, the biofeedback therapist may suggest that the person return to the attending physician for medication to facilitate the relaxation process. As symptoms improve, the need for some types of medicine, particularly analgesics or antianxiety meds, may decrease. With symptoms that require medication steadily decreasing, the person is encouraged to ask his or her physician to lessen the dosage of drugs or eliminate them altogether. In fact, the joint management of severe depression by the patient, physicians, biofeedback therapists, and CBT practitioners tends to be more the norm than the exception given the complexities of the existing health care system.

Biofeedback has not traditionally been recommended for people with major depressive disorder or chronic depression, although there are no contraindications or reports of the worsening of the depressive state with biofeedback. Depressed people experiencing chronic pain commonly experience a sense of helplessness regarding their pain and the limitations imposed by it. Biofeedback is based on the principle of gaining a sense of control over maladaptive physiological responses. The experience of success that results can be translated into a sense of self-control. During the course of therapy, this major nonspecific effect of biofeedback (i.e., developing a sense of more control over the physiological responses to stress) can facilitate learning how to control pain. Assessment of mood is important for the use of biofeedback for any chronic pain condition. Even if the severity of the mood disorder does not require psychiatric intervention, the nonspecific effects of biofeedback—more self-control—may be mobilized and directed toward improvement in both pain and mood. Anxiety is a frequent companion to chronic pain. Anxiety may present as the cognitive symptoms of fear of losing control, dying, or going crazy or as somatic symptoms such as racing heart, sweating, or shortness of breath. Appropriate candidates for biofeedback include those who suffer from clinical psychiatric illnesses, who can learn to modify specific physiological or psychological responses associated with their disorders. In school-age children readily identified as "anxious," significant reductions in situational and baseline anxiety can be achieved even at this early age with biofeedback.

Learning facial relaxation through biofeedback promotes lower nervous-system activity and can be effective in managing both the somatic and cognitive components of anxiety. Generalized anxiety disorder can also be treated in diagnosed adults. In terms of anxiety levels, the effects of biofeedback may be nonspecific, ranging from general relaxation to developing the insight and control necessary to overcome the disorder.

People with post-traumatic stress disorder (PTSD) another of the anxiety disorders, always requires therapy beyond biofeedback and relaxation. Some of the instigating causes of chronic pain are traumatic events, like personal assaults, war and combat, motor vehicle accidents, or serious work injury, and those who suffer from chronic pain should be evaluated for PTSD before initiating biofeedback treatment.

In the case of phobias, psychophysiological approaches including biofeedback and relaxation therapy are suggested as a first step in management, to be followed by medication if necessary. Relaxation therapy is integral to systematic desensitization, as gradual exposure to the phobic stimulus is combined with guided relaxation. Simultaneously, biofeedback can shorten the time required to learn relaxation under conditions of exposure to the phobic stimulus.

Syncope (fainting) can be a symptom of a simple phobia. For example, the sight of blood or injury can result in loss of consciousness in susceptible persons. In such a case electromyographic biofeedback and thermal biofeedback therapy can be combined with systematic desensitization—for example, with cognitive-behavioral therapy—to treat a long-standing blood/injury phobia. With therapy, the person learns to identify pre-fainting cues and to use biofeedback and relaxation techniques to block fainting when confronted with the phobic stimulus. Neurofeedback (i.e., EEG feedback), which is applied to the brain directly, has also been used successfully to treat anxiety disorders, particularly generalized anxiety and phobias.

Headache

Biofeedback is helpful for both tension-type and migraine headaches as well as for headaches that result from the overuse of medications and post-traumatic headaches (headaches that develop as a result of a head or brain injury). The headache sufferer is trained to decrease tension levels and produce a general relaxation response. Surface sensors are placed on the forehead to detect a wide range of muscular activity such as grimacing, frowning, and teeth clenching; learning to recognize these signals helps the person regulate muscle tension and thereby decrease pain. The relaxation process is then generalized to stressful situations where the person feels his muscles tensing or notices the early signs of a headache.

The most common biofeedback treatment for nondrug treatment of migraine headache is thermal biofeedback along with relaxation techniques. The results of this combination are comparable to those of the drug propranolol, a type of beta-blocker, and certainly are far superior to suffering through the headache and waiting it out. Long-term management of headache by means of biofeedback and relaxation therapy is effective when the person is able to learn to generalize the relaxation response to stressful situations and continue to use the adaptive coping techniques learned during the therapy.

Post-traumatic headache and headache due to high levels of drug consumption pose special challenges. Over half of these sufferers report at least moderate improvement in the number of headaches by using biofeedback, and nearly all show increased ability to relax and cope with the pain by using these same techniques. In general, however, the longer the duration of post-traumatic pain, the poorer the response. Headache sufferers who use high doses of multiple classes of medications are also challenging. Withdrawal of medication can be accomplished on an outpatient basis and, if possible, should precede biofeedback treatment. The active involvement of the therapist is critically important to success, rather than just having physicians passively writing and revoking prescriptions for pain medications.

Children and seniors are appropriate candidates for biofeedback therapy to treat chronic headache, although their reactions to it might be different. It is not necessarily the case that children learn to acquire biofeedback skills any faster than adults. Despite that fact, children's actual success rates with biofeedback are higher than those of adults, which may be because most children do not exhibit the companion depressive features so common in adults who struggle with daily headache pain. As well, young people are often intrigued by the biofeedback equipment, are comfortable with video game–type technology, and tend to adapt to the treatment setting quite easily. In contrast, older persons often require additional sessions and learn somewhat more slowly. Nonetheless, electromyographic biofeedback, which measures muscle tension, has been found to help decrease total headache activity and increase headache-free days in older persons.

Musculoskeletal Pain

People with chronic musculoskeletal pain as a result of different conditions or injuries often report a myriad of associated psychological and physical symptoms, including sleep disturbance, vague sensations of discomfort, anxiety, and depression. In such cases successful treatment must include interventions for each problem of the mind and body.

Chronic low-back pain, for example, requires a combined approach of biofeedback with physical therapy, exercise, correction of gait and posture, massage, and possibly shoe prosthetics.

Biofeedback is quite useful for training the person in general relaxation and in correcting specific muscle tension problems. It is important to monitor tension in postures other than reclining in a chair, because muscles automatically relax if the head is supported by a headrest. Poor posture, bracing by tensing the muscles, insomnia, and depression are often contributing or perpetuating factors in long-term pain. Electromyographic biofeedback is provided while in the sitting and/or standing positions. In addition, cognitive-behavioral therapy may be necessary to modify moods, thoughts, and behaviors. Follow-up sessions and relaxation practice are strongly recommended for maintaining improvement because relapse can occur after a person has learned the basic skills, particularly if lifestyle and posture have not changed.

Older people are good candidates for biofeedback treatment for chronic musculoskeletal pain. Mind-body therapies are as effective for older adults with pain as a result of osteoarthritis as they are for younger adults who have chronic pain or rheumatoid arthritis. Osteoarthritis and rheumatoid arthritis differ biologically but share the disability associated with pain and emotional distress. Biofeedback, along with progressive muscle relaxation or guided imagery (chapter 4), can achieve a 50 percent reduction in symptoms.

Fibromyalgia is a complex psycho-physiological disorder manifesting as muscle pain, tender points, and sleep disturbance. Many sufferers also report headache, fatigue, memory problems, anxiety, and depression. Environmental conditions such as changes in weather, noise level, and anything that interrupts sleep can often exacerbate the pain and discomfort. This chronic illness is severely distressing, and the physical symptoms are intensified by chronic stress, as the person who is already anxious is more aware of body pain and then becomes more anxious when feeling the pain. This is an example of an unhealthy, stressful, negative feedback loop. This pathologic process is particularly amenable to positive biofeedback. A 2001 study involving thirty patients with fibromyalgia syndrome who received biofeedback found that participants experienced statistically significant improvements in mental clarity, mood, and sleep.[4]

Management of fibromyalgia is a step-by-step process. The first step is making the right diagnosis. This has often been followed by starting a low dose of a tricyclic antidepressant at bedtime to break the cycle of insomnia, anxiety, and pain. These drugs are initially used to address depression, to restore sleep, and to break the cycle of pain and sleep disturbance, along with physical therapy and/or cognitive-behavioral therapy. The cognitive-behavioral therapy component is of major importance since more intense pain due to a low mood may be misinterpreted as a worsening of the syndrome. As well, there is good evidence for the efficacy of biofeedback for fibromyalgia, as mind-body therapy can be effective in increasing function, even if it does not specifically decrease pain. A change in the perception of pain can be accomplished after training with biofeedback

Treatment of chronic neck pain should ideally include patient education, relaxation, biofeedback, and cognitive-behavioral therapy. In such cases the person is educated as to how the pain signal is transmitted, learns to increase awareness of and thereby reduce neck-bracing response, and learns the muscular relaxation response. Cognitive-behavioral therapy is used to decrease the habitual negative moods and thoughts that impact the pain experience, including the maladaptive muscle contractions, together with biofeedback.

Phantom-limb pain following the traumatic amputation of a limb can be treated with biofeedback to reduce pain and modify the reorganization of nervous-system pain pathways in the brain that occur over time as a result of the experience of chronic pain. Chronic pain is partially a learned behavior. Repeated episodes of experiencing pain alter neuronal arrangements in the somatic and sensory cortex areas and memory areas of the brain. Operant conditioning and biofeedback may be used to help extinguish pain memories.

Sleep Disorders

Sleep disorders invariably accompany chronic pain as either a contributing cause of it or the result of it, in a self-reinforcing negative feedback loop. Categories of disturbed sleep that can be addressed by biofeedback include primary insomnia (one of the dyssomnias, or sleeping disorders involving difficulty getting to sleep, remaining asleep, or excessive sleepiness) and insomnia related to chronic pain. People with recurring, chronic pain report difficulties in initiating and maintaining sleep. A poor night's sleep results in daytime fatigue and problems functioning. In addition to disordered sleep as a consequence of pain and mood disorders, sleep deprivation that results from sleep interruptions (not simply fewer total hours) increases one's awareness of pain and may disrupt pain inhibitory mechanisms in the brain, thereby further aggravating the pain.

Sleep hygiene—a variety of different practices that are necessary to have normal, quality nighttime sleep and full daytime alertness—is essential and should be tried first. The following recommendations are relatively simple and provide a means of encouraging someone to take responsibility for healthful sleep (instead of relying on dangerous prescription medication): Try to go to bed at a regular hour before eleven p.m., do not use the computer in bed before going to sleep, avoid coffee and stimulants starting in the afternoon, don't drink alcohol to excess (no more than two drinks), lower the room temperature, and allow some fresh air (and oxygen) into the room. In addition, effective mind-body therapies for sleep disorders include progressive relaxation, cognitive-behavioral therapy, and stimulus control by avoiding extraneous noise, light, and activity.

Progressive relaxation facilitates improvements in shortening the time required for the onset of sleep, but evidence to date does not favor the use of biofeedback alone in cases of sleep disturbance in chronic pain situations. Stimulus control can be used to address situations when pain is associated with the bed or bedtime, when contemplating going to bed produces anxiety or stress over not being able to sleep instead of being associated with relaxation and drowsiness. Pain sufferers are encouraged to remove any stressful stimuli from the bedroom and recondition bedtime as a time for relaxation and mental quietude.

Vertigo and Balance

Behavioral-modification techniques have been successfully used with astronauts and pilots who demonstrate orthostatic intolerance (blood rushes to the feet upon standing) after exposure to zero or low gravity while in space. This suggests the application of biofeedback for vertigo and what is called "orthostatic hypotension," or feeling light-headed or fainting when standing up. Normally, when a person stands up, gravity draws blood down through the blood vessels, as in a standing column of fluid, to the legs and away from the head. Automatic reflexes adjust the flow of blood through the different blood vessels so that the blood supply is maintained to the head and upper body in the standing position. Without exposure to gravity, as in outer space, over time these automatic reflexes are attenuated or extinguished. Pilots have been trained in biofeedback techniques to increase blood pressure under supine and head-up tilt conditions. As well, autogenic therapy and biofeedback were applied to control motion sickness in otherwise healthy and well-conditioned astronauts. The protocol comprised training multiple physiological responses simultaneously for a total of six hours. Transfer of the responses learned in the laboratory were made to a variety of stimulus conditions, such as rotary chair, flight, and space shuttle flights.[5]

BOUNDARY TYPES: WHO BENEFITS AND WHY

As we have learned, the general goal of biofeedback therapy is to lower body tension and change negative reinforcement of biological patterns. Your ability to effect these types of biological changes is related to your emotional boundary type. Among the biological patterns of the different boundary types, note that biofeedback falls in the middle of the spectrum (remember, most people fall somewhere toward the middle of the spectrum, and not at the ends). As thick boundary types generally respond well to more *hands-on* approaches, biofeedback is especially suited to those with medium to thick boundary types. Biofeeback gives the thick boundary person—literally—data, information, and feedback to show that what is going in his or her body is really "real" and not "all in his/her head." But biofeedback is also broadly effective for a wide range of chronic conditions regardless of boundary type, appealing to thicker boundary individuals by putting them in charge, while benefiting thinner boundary people by providing visual validation of their feelings.

FINDING A PRACTITIONER

Biofeedback and relaxation therapy are techniques provided by various mental-health professionals and do not belong to any particular medical specialty or field of health care. They do not represent medical practice specialties or subspecialities, so you will be looking not for a "biofeedback therapist," but rather for a health practitioner who utilizes biofeedback.

In addition to being a mind-body technique of complementary and alternative medicine (CAM), biofeedback is used in many conventional health care disciplines, including internal medicine, dentistry, physical therapy and rehabilitation, psychology and psychiatry, and pain management. It is best but not always possible for the same practitioner to provide you with both psychotherapy and biofeedback. When a clinical psychologist, clinical counselor, social worker, or psychiatric nurse is also trained in biofeedback, single biofeedback treatment sessions can integrated with psychotherapy, hypnosis, or imagery. For example, you might spend the first half of a one-hour session in psychotherapy and the other half practicing biofeedback. On the other hand, your session might start with guided imagery–assisted biofeedback to create an atmosphere of trust between you and the therapist, followed by a session of psychotherapy. An experienced therapist can also help you manage any lack of motivation or uncertainty that might crop up.

4

Imagery and Visualization

Since humans first began contemplating the nature of the human experience, we have tried to define and explain the interior processes of the mind. Those experiences do not have any established physical referents, which is why philosophers have speculated for millennia on the nature of mental imagery.

In the twentieth century, scientists attempted to verify or measure these phenomena. In the 1920s, structural psychologists went so far as to say that mental images simply did not exist. This was summarized in the "imageless thought" theory, which stated that there is an objective significance that can be found within experiences that are not necessarily associated with specific words, symbols, or signs. William Wundt (1832–1920), the first person to ever call himself a psychologist, founded the first formal laboratory for psychological research in Leipzig, Germany. Wundt proposed three basic elements of consciousness: thoughts, perception, and feelings. He proposed that studying images would mean studying thought, since he believed that images coexist with thought. Yet Aristotle had long before asked the same question, "Is thought possible without imagery?" Evidence supporting the idea that imagery was not in fact required for thinking came in the late nineteenth century, when Sir Francis Galton (nephew of Charles Darwin) observed that people who had difficulty forming visual images were still capable of thinking. The later dominance of behaviorism between the 1920s and 1950s took imagery-based research out of mainstream psychology.

Since the cognitive psychology revolution of the 1960s, psychologists have done a great amount of work exploring and categorizing mental imagery and inner processes. Contemporary psychologists distinguish several types of imagery. The most common form that you routinely experience is memory. When you try to remember a place you used to live, the furniture in your old house, or what the seats of your old car felt like, you immediately and necessarily conjure up a visual image in your mind—or in the "mind's eye." This is referred to as "forming a mental picture." Some people believe that they do not actually see or visualize the scene; rather, they simply have a strong sense of the scene and know what it looks and feels like.

WHAT IS IMAGERY?

Imagery is defined as "pictures of people or things in a work of art"; it also refers to "language that causes people to imagine pictures in their mind." As well, it describes a wide array of procedures used in therapy to encourage a person to change ingrained attitudes, behaviors, or physiological reactions. As a mental process, imagery is associated with sensory qualities, or re-creating sensations in perception. In addition to the visual sense (sight/seeing), this includes all the other senses: aural (sound/hearing), tactile (touch), olfactory (smell), proprioceptive (position or orientation), and kinesthetic (movement).

Imagery is frequently used synonymously with *visualization*. However, visualization refers only to "seeing" something in the mind's eye, whereas imagery is a broader category and usually involves one sense or a combination of senses producing an image. Thus imagery goes beyond visualization to essentially include "imaging" any sensory perception. Mental scanning, a technique developed by American psychologist and neuroscientist Stephen Kosslyn, is a technique that has been used to support the depictive theory of imagery; in this method you create mental images and then scan them in your mind. Kosslyn was one of the first to introduce theories in both imagery and perception (i.e., perceptual images that we actually see with our own eyes).

To show that we use the same spatial mechanisms in the brain in imagery as we do in visual perception, Kosslyn formed this experiment: He asked participants to memorize a picture of an object and then to create an image of that object in their mind and to focus on one particular part of it. The participants were then asked to look for another part of the object in their mental image and press a "yes" button when they found the new part of the object or a "no" button if they couldn't find it at all. Kosslyn wanted to observe whether or not participants took longer to find parts of the object located farther from the initial part they had focused on. If not, it would mean they were scanning across the entire object as a whole. Kosslyn's research in imagery continued for over a decade and it was a lot more complicated than he had foreseen (perhaps in his mind's eye). He eventually arrived at new insights and formed the conclusion that imagery, like perception, is served by a spatial mechanism, and that these same mechanisms are shared with perception. This helps us see the significance of how our perceptual mechanisms are interlinked with imagery mechanisms in the same location in the brain.

Memory Enhancement Techniques

Imagery seems to have attracted attention during early mnemonic experiences in ancient Greece. A mnemonic device is, of course, a pattern of letters, ideas, or associations that assist us in remembering something. It was discovered by the Greek poet and *sophos* (wise man) Simonides (ca. 556–468 BCE). Supposedly, Simonides was asked by the gods to go outside a banquet hall located in Thessaly, whereupon he recited a poem. While he was briefly outside the hall conversing with the gods, the roof collapsed, crushing the people inside beyond recognition. Later he was able to identify corpses whose features were otherwise impossible to recognize by using his memory of where the people had been situated around the banquet table when he left the party. Thus, what is known as the "method of loci" was initiated (in Latin, *locus* is a location; *loci* is the plural form), which refers to the method of memory enhancement that uses visualization along with the use of spatial memory (like Kosslyn's experiments above) and familiar information about one's environment to quickly and efficiently recall information. Simonides stated that people must select places and form mental images of the things they wish to remember, and then store those images so the order of the places will preserve the order of things.[1]

Another device related to visualization is the mnemonic peg system, a memory aid that works by creating mental associations between two concrete objects in a one-to-one fashion that will later be applied to to-be-remembered information. The ancient Greek god of knowledge, medicine, and music, Apollo, was said in legend to have laid out the groundwork for this system. However, it is the sixteenth-century English "professor of the art of memory" Henry Herdson who is credited for inventing this system, which typically involves linking nouns to numbers. It is common practice to choose a noun that rhymes with the number with which it is associated, such as *gun* for 1, *shoe* for 2, *tree* for 3, *door* for 4, *hive* for 5, and so forth. These associations become the pegs of the system. The last step is to associate the number-word with a vivid visual image. These elements are more easily remembered if you can tap into your emotional body to create a visceral connection that uses images. The rule of short-term memory is that the average person can memorize up to seven digits (thus the original practice of using seven digits for phone numbers); anything more is too much for the short-term memory to hold. The peg system was designed to overcome this tendency.

The Brain, Perception, and Imagery

The examples provided above are based purely on empirical observations when it comes to memory capacity. What is actually going on in the brain has only become "visible" using new brain imaging techniques. These new studies show us what individual neurons in the brain "light up" when we use our perceptual vision (receiving information through the eyes) versus using our imaginations. Scientists have discovered that when a person visually perceives an object, the neurons respond similarly as when that person images the same object.[2] This was shown in 2004, when researchers used functional magnetic resonance imaging (functional MRI) to detect areas of activity in the brain underlying visual mental imagery and visual perception. The brain scans, which showed activation in the frontal lobe for perception and imagery, were almost identical for both.[3] There was slightly more activity in the perceptual tasks, since the frontal lobe is the location of the visual receiving area. As light enters the eyes in the retina, impulses then travel along the optic nerve to reach the visual cortex in the occipital lobe.

Dream Images

Creating images with the mind and in the mind offers a way of communicating with the subconscious and the unconscious (deeper-than-conscious) aspects of the self. This kind of communication becomes apparent when considering the dream state. Dreams communicate mainly in images, which are then consciously interpreted to make a story. While Sigmund Freud made a name for himself as a psychotherapist with his 1900 book *The Interpretation of Dreams,* you can fundamentally interpret your own dreams better than any psychoanalyst because it is your own unconscious mind that serves up the various vivid images that arise in dreams. The conscious aspects of your mind then automatically work to string them together into some kind of coherent narrative (assuming you can remember the images at all once you wake up).

Dreams occur during the fifth stage of sleep, called REM, the phase of rapid eye movement. We tend to go into REM sleep more frequently and deeply as the morning approaches. Interestingly, the body behaves as if it were awake during REM sleep—typically, in this state the brain produces the same beta waves as it does when you are awake and demonstrates psychological, physiological, and biochemical activity as well. REM sleep also involves theta waves. These work in the hippocampal region of the brain to improve short-term memory processes.[4] When you don't get enough sleep, your prefrontal cortex, responsible for problem solving and alertness, decreases in performance. This area of the brain is also in charge of proper mental functioning in both simple and complex tasks and processing working or short-term memory (which is similar to random-access memory on your personal computer)—what you need in order to eventually retain information in the long term. Long-term memory is affected when you do not get enough hours of sleep at night. You should try to get adequate sleep every night, as trying to "catch up" by sleeping in on the weekends doesn't replenish the brain in the same way. For new information composed of short-term memory to be retained as long-term memory, that information needs to be processed within twenty-four hours and we need the rest of our sleeping hours to complete this process. If you don't get enough sleep (including REM sleep), your ability to hold images in the mind decreases.

The Communicative Quality of Imagery

Imagery is essentially a way of thinking that accesses sensory capabilities and functions in the absence of sensory input. It can be considered one of brain's higher-order encoding systems. The system that you are probably most familiar with is called the sequential information-processing system. This underlies linear, analytic, and conscious verbal thinking, which is typically associated with the left hemisphere of the brain ("left-brain thinking"). Most medical and scientific professionals, for example, must come up through an educational system where they become highly educated and are highly rewarded for their abilities using this limited mode of information processing. Imagery, on the other hand, is a language utilized by a simultaneous information-processing mode that underlies the holistic, synthetic, pattern thinking of the unconscious mind, which is typically associated with the right hemisphere of the brain ("right-brain thinking").

The communicative quality of imagery is important because feelings and behaviors evoked by images are primarily motivated by subconscious and unconscious factors. Because it often involves directed concentration, imagery can also be regarded as another form of guided meditation or relaxation (see chapter 2). In fact, many practices discussed in the first few chapters of this book use a component of imagery. Psychotherapy, hypnosis, and biofeedback all use various elements of it. Any therapy that relies on the mental imagination (another term for imagery) to stimulate, communicate, solve problems, or evoke a heightened awareness or sensitivity may be considered a form of imagery.

A Language of the Emotions

Imagery is a language of the arts, but it is also very much a language of the emotions. Emotions reveal what is important to us; they can be either potent motivators, getting us into gear, or barriers to changing lifestyle and habits. The emotions are also very much tied to physiological changes in the body, including varying patterns of muscle tension, blood flow, respiration, metabolism, and neurologically and immunologically active peptide secretions. What you "feel" of your emotions is also determined by your personality boundary or emotional type—thick or thin.

Modern research in the field of psychoneuroimmunology, the study of the interaction between psychological processes and the nervous and immune systems of the human body, points to the emotions as key modulators of neurologically active peptides secreted by the brain, gut, and immune system. Imagery relates to cognition, emotion, and physiology and can be considered a code or connection in mind-body interactions. Imagery also has direct physiological consequences and effects. In the absence of competing sensory cues, the body responds to imagery as it would to a genuine external experience. Emotionally engaged imagery has been shown in numerous research studies to be able to affect almost all major physiological control systems of the body—respiration, heart rate, blood pressure, metabolic rates in cells, gastrointestinal mobility and secretion, sexual function, and immune response. The numerous studies that have been done on mental imagery reveal that it

- influences oxygen supply in tissues;[5]
- brings about changes in cardiovascular,[6] vascular, and thermal regulation;[7]
- affects the pupillary and cochlear reflexes;[8]
- affects heart rate and galvanic skin responses;[9] and
- stimulates salivation.[10]

A case study related to us by Dr. Marty Rossman, an international expert and early pioneer in the use of guided imagery, illustrates the importance of engaging the emotions in guided imagery work. A sixty-year-old woman with metastatic cancer and chronic pain was having difficulty creating mental images of her immune system vigorously fighting her tumor. Cancer patients are often asked to form images of their own immune system cells (white blood cells) eating their cancer cells or fighting the cancer in some other way. However, this woman's imagery consisted of a few relatively inert immune cells sitting on the tumor, which she described as a "blob." Numerous therapeutic interventions failed to increase the immune activity she imagined. Finally her guide asked her to allow her mind to form an image of anything that was interfering with her ability to more actively visualize her healing. An image of a large chasm came to her mind. Across the chasm she saw her husband and grown children waving for her to come over. She began to cry at this image, the first evidence of emotion evidenced in many sessions. She explained that her family was emotionally distant and estranged from one another. In her imagery she wanted to build a bridge over to them (she was an engineer by training). She was encouraged to imagine building the bridge and walking across, into the welcoming arms of her embracing family. As a result of this session she became determined to ask her family to meet together with a family therapist, something they had never done. After a short series of deeply moving therapy sessions, the family members bonded in ways they never had before. Subsequently, the woman's healing imagery became very vigorous and active, as did her participation in other aspects of her treatment, including nutrition, exercise, and an experimental clinical trial of monoclonal antibodies.[11]

With her guide's encouragement, this woman was able to access, experience, and overcome an emotional barrier to her being more participatory in her own healing. Her imagery had not only cognitive but also emotional information that she was able to process in a nonlinear but meaningful way that led to action and to her eventual recovery.

Using Imagery to Relieve Chronic Pain

Imagery is a natural part of the way you think. It can almost always be helpful in a virtually unlimited number of situations for people with chronic pain. There are three major ways that imagery is used to address chronic pain:

1. Relaxation and stress-reduction techniques are necessarily a component of imagery work, as you can't do it unless you're in a relatively relaxed state. Relaxation is easy to teach, easy to learn, and almost universally helpful in alleviating pain. An imagery session typically begins with some form of relaxation, using any of the techniques described in chapter 2.

2. Visualization, or directed imagery, encourages you to imagine desired outcomes in a relaxed state of mind. This approach can be compared to cognitive-behavioral therapy, where the client is encouraged to go out with a new frame of mind and build a fund of positive new experiences as a reservoir of good, or better, feelings about life. With directed imagery you actually imagine these positive experiences occurring to you, and you begin to benefit from positive feelings before they actually occur in reality. But to the mind and to the body, as indicated by the body's responses, the fund of positive feelings is real. This approach also affords you a sense of participation and control in your own healing, which is of significant value. In addition, it may well relieve or reduce pain symptoms, stimulate healing responses in the body, and provide effective motivation for making positive life changes. Guided imagery works directly on the brain's perception of pain.

3. Receptive, or insight-oriented, imagery is where the images you form are invited into your conscious awareness and explored ("interpreted") in order to gather more information about a pain symptom, underlying illness, mood, situation, or solution. This approach is more like traditional psychotherapy, without all the Freudian baggage. Instead, you focus on your current experiences and feelings (instead of your past feelings about your mother, for example).

GUIDED IMAGERY: HOW IT WORKS

The term *guided imagery* describes a range of techniques, from simple visualization and directed imagery–based suggestion to metaphor and storytelling. Interactive guided imagery refers to a particular approach to using guided imagery in a therapeutic setting in which images are evoked from the person by a guide who, rather than suggesting specific images, interacts with the person to discover what is unique to him or her, helping to draw the appropriate images out. In this way, interactive guided imagery provides the person with a way to draw on his or her own inner resources to support healing, to make appropriate adaptations to changes in health, and to find creative solutions to challenges that were previously thought to be insoluble. The interactive process encourages the person to access his or her own strengths and resources, which leads to greater autonomy and self-efficacy and a sense of control over outcomes.

As an example, visualizing having a conversation with an imaginary figure that is both wise and loving—say, an inner healer—can be facilitated with the help of an experienced guide. The inner healer is characterized by qualities of wisdom and compassion (in analytic psychotherapy the term used is *ego ideal*). As the client is invited to imagine a figure that has these qualities, an exploration of whatever image arises out of the person's own mind can be meaningful and helpful in the sense that the inner healer can provide a way to access one's own inner wisdom and compassion. These qualities are beneficial in addressing and treating chronic pain.

In interactive guided imagery, the use of highly evocative images can help shift one's mood and mental state. By engaging the emotions, this type of imagery allows new behaviors and insights to become more accessible. Through the use of memory, fantasy, and sensory information, the guide encourages you to identify a personal quality or qualities that would serve especially well in your current situation. Highly evocative imagery helps you access the strengths you already have, to help you make the best use of your innate healing abilities.

The key to the effectiveness of interactive guided imagery is the *interactive* component. By working closely with the person instead of just passively reading from a canned imagery script, the guide ensures that the experience has personal meaning for the client and that the work proceeds at a pace determined by that person's unique needs and abilities. The guide uses nonjudgmental, content-free language because it encourages the client to tap into his or her own inner resources to find solutions for solving problems. Because both the content and the direction are set by the client, it is ultimately the client who sits in the driver's seat, guiding the process toward the resources needed to support healing, change, and positive therapeutic results, while the guide serves as a facilitator.

The following case study that illustrates how interactive guided imagery works was again related to us by Dr. Marty Rossman. A twenty-seven-year-old man with chronic pain was invited to allow an image to come to mind that represented his pain. But rather than encountering an image that was frightening, he found that a benign spirit image appeared. The man was encouraged by the guide to imagine that he could communicate with the image, and that it could communicate back to him in a way he could understand. When he asked the image what it wanted from him, it said, to his surprise, "You are a spiritual being, but there is no room for me in your life. Make room for me to live or I will have to return with you to the world of the spirits." The man cried and talked at length about his own spiritual seeking as an adolescent and young adult. Some years before his pain diagnosis he had become very involved in a lucrative business that had consumed all his waking hours. As a result he had gotten divorced and had lost many friends. Following the interactive experience of working with this inner guide over the course of treatment, he was able to change his priorities, and he subsequently went through a successful treatment for his pain. A much more balanced life resulted, including more time for friends, a spiritual practice, and philanthropic work, all of which stemmed from that initial encounter with his own healing spirit.[12]

Note that if this particular image had been directly suggested by the guide, the man might not have been able to relate. But by pulling this image out of himself rather than having someone else do it for him, the man was empowered to become aware of his own unconscious needs, which were directly related to his illness, his pain, and his ultimate healing and lifestyle changes. This case provides an example of a term that crops up frequently in interactive guided imagery: *the higher self.* The higher self is an intelligence that is a part of you but is not part of your everyday thinking. The presence of the higher self is usually indicated when a person receives a download of information that leads to deep insights, such as what this man experienced.

Creating a Healing Space in Your Mind's Eye

A guided imagery session typically begins with abdominal breathing, followed by a simple body scan, or progressive muscle relaxation. You are then invited to imagine being in a beautiful, safe place you love to be in. Depending on the person and the guide, this might also be called a "healing place" or a "place of power." In any case, safety is always a critical factor. It may be a place that you know and have been to before, either in real life or in your imagination, or a new place might come to mind. When being guided using an interactive approach, you might be invited to describe the place where you imagine yourself. The guide asks you what you see, hear, and feel there, allowing you to respond. Questions like "What time of day does it seem to be there?" and "What is the weather like there?" can help you focus on having a visceral, emotional experience and deepen the subjective reality of the imagery.

As simple as this technique is, it illustrates the utility of the interaction between the guided and the guide. The guide might suggest that you imagine yourself at a beautiful beach with warm sun and sand and bluish-green waves breaking on the shore. While this setting works well for most people, it may be that for some reason that image doesn't work for you. For instance, perhaps you were particularly affected by watching the movie *Jaws* or had a near-drowning experience as a child, and this kind of setting brings up fear. For this reason there is everything to gain by making this a truly interactive process between the guided and the guide. Certainly, if you are being guided to go to a place of your choice that is beautiful, safe, and relaxing, you will invariably pick a place that fulfills those criteria.

Ideal Model Imaging

Imagery consists of more than just visualizing. Although vision is a dominant sense for humans, it is only one of five. There may also be sounds of healing (common in shamanic healing in traditional cultures), a fragrance (as in essential oils therapy), or body sensations such as warmth, coolness, or tingling that accompany your healing imagery. You will be encouraged to explore all the senses in creating and elaborating on your personal healing imagery. Functional MRIs have shown that as people imagine different senses, different areas of the cerebral cortex are activated in the brain. Recruiting different senses and more cortical areas of the brain is likely to make the imagery more subjectively real and more powerfully stimulating of the subcortical responses that mediate healing and immune-system function.

In ideal model imagery you develop imagery around what you consider to be the ideal outcome to encourage this reality. This can consist of ideal personality attributes or character traits that you admire and would like to express yourself, or what it will be like when you recover your health and overcome your pain. You might imagine doing what you love doing, with the people you love doing it with, enjoying landmark events such as family weddings, births, graduations, promotions, and other significant life events, or reaching goals such as renewed independence. Ideal model imagery is not always easy, and it may bring up significant barriers to investing hope in recovery, but this then allows you to work with those potential barriers. As well, ideal model imagery can bring up grief. You can simply acknowledge and process as much or as little as needed until you can imagine your desired goal as an intended direction, without the grief. Visualization can be a powerful tool for combating chronic pain, cancer, infection, and other illnesses, provided the imagery is guided by someone with expertise and ethics. However, visualizing certain outcomes under the wrong circumstances, with insufficiently trained people as guides, can actually lead to a decline in motivation and less possibility for the ultimate achievement of a goal if visualizers feel like they have already achieved their objectives. For example, among today's proliferation of so-called management gurus, it has been observed that by jumping the gun they can make everyone feel good in the workplace before they have even accomplished anything. This kind of ham-handed approach actually takes away from productivity and undermines the resolution of real problems by providing people with psychic rewards before they have achieved any real results. This kind of universal trophy-for-everybody mentality has affected our entire modern culture and society. On the other hand, competent practitioners of guided imagery, by combining the benefits of optimism with the pragmatic survival skills of realism, can create a healthy balance without emphasizing unrealistic or unrealized expectations. As well, being able to visualize the worst-case scenario actually reduces anxiety levels. When you can assess how bad things can possibly get, you usually discover ways that you could cope (and usually things never get that bad anyway).

Related to ideal model imaging is what is known as the "nocebo effect." Most people know about the placebo effect, which relates to the healing power of positive intentions and expectations (thereby tapping into the body's own potent self-healing potential). The nocebo effect, in contrast, relates to having poor expectations that lead to poor health outcomes. This component is especially important if people have heard or experienced negative messages about their prognosis from their doctors, whether communicated intentionally or unintentionally. For example, when participants in a clinical drug trial are informed about all the possible side effects of a treatment, they may actually experience them—even if they're given the placebo rather than the drug itself. In fact, many people drop out of studies due to the nocebo effect. For example, 11 percent of the placebo group in one recent fibromyalgia study dropped out, while in statin (cholesterol) drug trials, nocebo-related dropout rates ranged from 4 to 26 percent.[13]

Many patients say something like "I will never forget the look on my doctor's face when he told me I would have to learn to live with my pain" or report their doctor saying "There is really nothing we can do." A doctor's choice of words has important consequences for a patient's state of mind and expectations. Dr. Bernard Lown, the original developer of the direct-current defibrillator and the cardioverter as well as a recipient of the Nobel Peace Prize, was also the pioneer of nonsurgical treatments for heart disease and the originator of the concept of "avoidable care." He says, "Words are the most powerful tool a doctor possesses, but words, like a two-edged sword, can maim as well as heal."

For example, in one study, when given pain-relieving injections prior to surgery, patients felt better when they were told it would make the procedure go better, but they felt worse when warned that the injection would hurt.[14] In these days of risk management and informed consent, doctors may feel compelled to recite a long litany of everything that could possibly go wrong and all the negative side effects a patient might experience. Simply telling patients all this makes them feel worse, and informing them about side effects often increases the likelihood that they will actually experience them—the power of suggestibility that has a net negative effect. This problem, of course, poses an ethical dilemma. For your (or your doctor's) own peace of mind, though, your local hospital might now have a professional medical ethicist on staff—yet another medical subspecialty that has been minted due to our overspecialized, dysfunctional mainstream health care system.

We tend to not really want our doctors to be just regular people; we want them to be potent and powerful healers and helpers, somewhat like ideal parents. Verbal and nonverbal cues from doctors can create anxiety, depression, or even a kind of post-traumatic stress syndrome resulting in intrusive thinking, sleep disturbance, excessive vigilance, and anxiety. This kind of situation is especially difficult to address and often requires much attention to neutralize or negate. One way to begin to go about doing this is to imagine being in the doctor's office, with a calendar on the wall, with a future date that is meaningful to you, imagining the doctor reviewing your test results and giving you good news, and you feeling elated. This is an image that you can substitute for the one you might have unconsciously adopted due to a doctor's careless comments and provides a way for you to respond in a more internally effective manner.

Visualizing Pain and Its Opposite

One way to use visualization to heal chronic pain is to create an image that characterizes the area of pain, then create a second image to counteract that pain image. For example, the pain might be seen as a flashing red light; the counteracting image might be a descending angel who overcomes the light with a warm, suffusing glow. Once this image is formulated, the person uses a relaxation or meditation technique to access the levels where his or her self-healing power resides and then imagines a picture of healing with a warm, glowing light illuminating a future free of pain. This process may be repeated in sessions with the guide as often as necessary, allowing for changes to the healing image that might spontaneously occur either or in response to a change in the image of pain. Again, when a person repeatedly imagines him- or herself as having already achieved a desired goal—the healing image—the deeper mind gradually accepts this new image and works to bring it into reality.

Moving from Insight to Action

Grounding, which may literally involve connecting your energy to the geophysical energy of the earth, is a process by which the insights evoked in imagery are turned into actions. Your new awareness and motivation are then focused into a specific plan for attitudinal, emotional, or behavioral change. This process of adding the will to the imagination involves clarification of insights, brainstorming, choosing the best option, affirmations, action planning, imagery rehearsal, and constant reformulation ("rebooting") of the plan until it actually succeeds. Connecting a new awareness to a specific action is often the missing link in image therapy. Imagery can be used to enhance this process by providing creative options for action and allowing troubleshooting and practice through rehearsal. This process can actually help you change your dietary and exercise habits and reduce stress by resolving problems that you previously were unable to resolve.

When you have an out-of-body experience, you may find you are in an unpleasant state, feeling a buzzing, dissonant energy that comes from not connecting with your physical, mental, and emotional levels. A buzzing or dissonance can also occur from things like working on a computer for hours without a break, or working by rote, without being fully in the present moment. Ungroundedness is an uneasy energy within yourself. Being ungrounded can feel as if there is a buzzing sensation in or toward the top of your head. Being ungrounded can mean that you are not thinking clearly and you feel high-strung and nervous, temperamental, or unstable. When you connect to yourself and your own awareness of yourself, insights can come through much more easily. For instance, strong concentration on mental images will help you connect to yourself more deeply, inspiring powerful change. Imagine an image with the power to light your path to better self-awareness, setting aside the pain.

For example, if you imagine yourself in a better life circumstance than you have been in by focusing on positive emotions such as love, harmony, and positive connection with yourself and others, you will deepen these feelings in reality by first experiencing them in the imagination. By imagining, you are focusing on specific feelings and the thoughts that may come along with these feelings. You will then start making appropriate and positive life decisions that will continue to deepen these feelings and thoughts in reality. Daily meditation with strong visualizations can foster change because you are reprogramming your way of feeling *and* thinking. Thus, the actions and decisions that follow suit will be in accordance with the thoughts and feelings you experience during meditation and visualization.

THE PROVEN EFFECTIVENESS OF IMAGERY

In recent years there have been thousands of studies done on using imagery as an effective healing modality. It is not uncommon to find it in many different health settings today, and in particular it has gained wide acceptance in the field of nursing.

Anxiety and Depression
A 2002 community-based study conducted in Sydney, Australia, involved people with advanced cancer who were experiencing anxiety and depression. Participants in the study were randomly assigned to one of four treatment options: (1) progressive muscle relaxation training; (2) guided imagery training; (3) both of the preceding; and (4) a control group that used none of these treatment options. Throughout the study, participants were tested for anxiety, depression, and quality of life. There was no significant improvement for anxiety for the methods tested, but significant positive changes for depression and overall quality of life were observed.[15] Guided imagery, as seen in multiple studies including the one

just mentioned, is able to take people out of their current state and, based on their level of imagination, completely replace their current state with a more positive or productive outlook and state of being.

Surgery (Before and After)

Nurses at a community hospital in Pennsylvania found that providing their patients with guided imagery CDs proved effective in a variety of ways. The guided imagery recordings helped patients relieve pain and anxiety before and after surgery, helped them relax and sleep better during their hospital stay, helped lower blood pressure, and reduced the need for breathing and respiratory devices. The nurses also reported that the guided imagery CDs were often more effective than sedation for easing confusion in older patients. Each bedside contained a packet of CDs and a CD player with earphones. Each of the CDs focused on a major component of a successful hospital stay—for example, health and healing, comfort, peaceful rest, courage, and serenity. In addition to providing patients with these guided imagery recordings, all the staff nurses, therapists, social workers, and managers were trained in the use of the guided imagery CDs, and many used them themselves for their personal benefit.[16]

Another study was conducted in 1993 to compare the effectiveness of various types of guided imagery for preoperative patients. Three outcomes were examined: intraoperative blood loss (blood loss during surgical procedures), length of hospital stay, and use of postoperative pain medication. A population of 335 surgical patients were randomly assigned to five groups. Each of the four experimental groups was provided with a guided imagery audiotape created by four different therapists. The control group received an audiotape with a "whooshing" noise. The results of this study showed that three of the four audiotapes produced no significant benefits on any of the medical outcomes examined, while the control group also registered no benefits on the medical outcomes. By contrast, the guided-imagery audiotape, produced by Belleruth Naparstek, a highly regarded therapist and imagery practitioner, produced highly significant results in two outcomes, blood loss and length of stay. Naparstek's tape was much more sophisticated than the others. Her imagery had been scored with specially composed music designed to highlight and accompany each image, with an emphasis on spiritual connectedness. Naparstek included visualizations of positive outcomes, fast wound healing, less pain, and no nausea.[17]

Cleveland Clinic researchers measured 130 colorectal surgery patients for anxiety levels, pain perceptions, and narcotic medication requirements. The treatment group listened to guided imagery tapes for three days prior to surgery, as well as during anesthesia induction, intra-operatively, after anesthesia, and for six days after surgery. The controls received routine preoperative care. Patients in the guided imagery group experienced considerably less preoperative and postoperative anxiety and pain, and they required 50 percent less narcotic medication after surgery than the controls.[18]

BOUNDARY TYPES: WHO BENEFITS AND WHY

As seen in the boundary-type diagram on page 20, guided imagery falls around the midpoint line of boundary types, leaning slightly toward thick emotional types. People on the thin side of the boundary spectrum are often better able to identify their feelings compared to people on the thick side. Based on this, we could project that thin boundary types may also respond well to guided imagery and visualization. Thus guided imagery may be useful in alleviating *both* thick and thin boundary conditions.

FINDING A PRACTITIONER

Many health professionals use guided imagery in their work, although quite a few may have only limited training, where they've learned only by leading someone through noninteractive scripts. The quality of this type of intervention is questionable. Because there is potential for doing more harm than good when these techniques are used inappropriately or by someone without adequate skills, standards of practice and quality control are important criteria in choosing a practitioner. The Academy for Guided Imagery is a postgraduate training institution founded in 1989 to bring quality standards to the training of imagery practitioners. Certification by this organization is largely based on a training program that involves direct observation of clinical work in small-group and individually supervised sessions. Each candidate is observed by four to six different faculty members during their fifty-two hours of training that leads to certification. You can find an imagery guide in your area at their website, www.acadgi.com.

There are various considerations in using imagery effectively as a self-care technique, in a group or class, or as part of an individual counseling or therapy relationship. Self-help books and tapes are an inexpensive option if you are able to use these techniques on your own. Oftentimes people explore all of these options and choose the one(s) best suited to them and to the nature of their pain condition, the coping responses, and the personal approaches to healing, as well as the amount of time, energy, and funds you are willing or able to invest in the process. However, effectively dealing with highly charged emotional issues often requires the assistance of a competent professional imagery guide.

In addition to possessing adequate training in imagery work, imagery guides should bring certain personal qualities to the therapeutic experience, including a nonjudgmental attitude, patience, and trust in the client's own abilities to bring about healing. A guide is a facilitator; he or she should always be cognizant that it is the client's own resources that provide strength and solutions. Moreover, when the client believes in his or her own internal resources, it is far less likely that he or she will rely only on therapists. This approach provides optimal opportunities for effective self-care, an enhanced sense of self-control, and the rapid development of independence.

In terms of frequency, we do not know the "dose-response" relationship of healing imagery, even though we know that it has a positive effect. Most studies have used protocols of twenty minutes, two or three times a day. Studies indicate that the more people do imagery practices, the more they benefit, whether due to the practice itself or because intensive practice simply serves as a marker of the intention to treat, the determination to help, and the belief that it will succeed. People are encouraged to think frequently about their healing imagery, even if only for a few seconds, and especially whenever they do anything they hope or think will help their healing, like taking medications, vitamins, herbs, or other treatments. At the same time we are encouraged to take time at least once during the day to relax, shift our attention, and focus on nothing but the healing process, however we might imagine it.

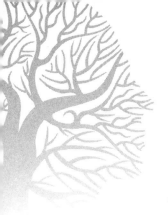

5
Hypnosis

Hypnosis has earned a secure place in modern medicine in the treatment of pain, even though it has had a somewhat controversial history. Despite its enduring mysterious quality and its regular use in some rather unscientific venues, health practitioners have maintained a continued interest in its use for a long time. Communication with the unconscious had been exclusively the domain of hypnosis until guided imagery, relaxation, and other mind-body techniques emerged in more recent years. A completely noninvasive approach that harnesses your body's own power to heal itself, hypnosis joins these other modalities to earn a well-deserved place in modern medicine. It can accomplish truly remarkable results and is one of the best treatment options out there—provided you are susceptible to hypnosis, which is related to your personality boundary or emotional type.

Hypnosis emerged in the late eighteenth century with Austrian physician Franz Anton Mesmer, whose development of the first experiments in hypnosis arose out of his theory that a universal magnetic "fluid" existed in all living beings, and that disease or pain resulted when this fluid was out of balance. Hypnosis didn't find its way into mainstream medical practice until the 1950s, however.

Since then, interest in hypnosis has grown, and its practice has found numerous clinical applications, including (and especially) pain management. The technique is important for various psychological and medical conditions and has been used successfully to treat everything from anxiety to helping people quit smoking. It has also found important applications in the treatment of such varied disorders as migraine headache, irritable bowel syndrome, and sleep disorders, as well as in the relief of chronic and acute pain.[1] In fact, hypnosis appears to be a promising tool for many kinds of physical ailments.

With the advent of sophisticated brain-imaging techniques such as MRI and PET scanning, it has been possible for the first time to understand some of the physiological changes that occur during and as a result of a hypnotic state—proving beyond a shadow of a doubt that hypnosis is very much for real.

THE HISTORY OF HYPNOSIS

The origins of hypnosis as a distinctive medical practice are found in the colorful career of Franz Anton Mesmer (1734–1815), a charismatic and controversial figure. Mesmer developed theories involving "animal magnetism," which he defined as a natural energetic transference that occurred among all animate and inanimate objects, as well cosmic bodies, as in astrology and the effects of planetary tides on the body's gravitational forces.[2] He used trancelike states and the power of suggestion in treating his patients, giving rise to the popular term *mesmerize*. Mesmer did not ask questions, but he did make suggestions. He developed a large European clientele as a result of his success in helping people gain improvements in their symptoms. His ideas, however, were judged radical even in light of the eighteenth-century interest in vitalism, which proposed that "living organisms are fundamentally different from non-living entities because they contain some non-physical element or are governed by different principles than are inanimate things."[3]

Controversy surrounding Mesmer's work led him to leave Austria for France, where King Louis XVI ordered a commission to be assembled in Paris to evaluate Mesmer's work. This assembly included such medical and scientific luminaries as the chemist Antoine Lavoisier (who was soon to lose his head, together with King Louis and Marie Antoinette) and Joseph Guillotine (the inventor of the "humane" execution apparatus, which was used on those above and many others in revolutionary France), as well as the newly appointed American ambassador to France, Benjamin Franklin. The panel initially designed experiments that would have provided a fair scientific evaluation, but it soon degenerated into arguments about hypnosis's mechanisms of action—which have not yet been resolved to this day. The outcome was not favorable to Mesmer's ideas. It was concluded by King Louis's panel that any apparent benefit of Mesmer's technique was the work of the imagination, and he was ultimately labeled a fraud and driven into exile in Germany, where his exact activities during the last twenty years of his life are largely unknown. However, Mesmer had discovered the power that suggestion using mental imagery had for modifying somatic symptoms such as pain. One of his students, Dr. Charles D'Elson, commented after the Louis XVI committee report, "If Mesmer has no other secret than that he has been able to make the imagination exert an influence upon health, would he not still be a wonder doctor? If treatment by the use of the imagination is the best treatment, why do we not make use of it?"[4] It's a good question, and one that still resonates today.

Interest in mesmerism was rekindled in the 1840s, when British surgeons employed hypnotic techniques in their clinical practices. It was at that time that the term *hypnotism,* from the Greek *hypnos,* "sleep," was coined by the English surgeon James Braid. He realized that hypnosis was a result not of external forces, but of the subject's ability to summon his or her own powers of focus and concentration.[5]

An influential nineteenth-century practitioner of hypnosis for surgical anesthesia was the Scottish surgeon James Esdaile. In the era just before chemical anesthetics like nitrous oxide and ether were available, Esdaile used hypnosis as the sole method of anesthesia in over three hundred major operations and received widespread notice in Europe and the United States. With a relatively low mortality rate for these surgical procedures, Esdaile's efforts lent respectability to the clinical practice of hypnosis. However, soon chemical anesthetic agents began to be used, following Boston dentist William Thomas Green Morton's successful 1846 demonstration to medical students at Massachusetts General Hospital, in which he used diethyl ether. Ether quickly supplanted hypnosis for surgical anesthesia because it was easier to use and took less time to administer (although it was not as safe).

During the late nineteenth century, hypnosis was revived in France as a result of the interest in the newly developing fields of psychiatry and psychology. At that time, neuropathologists were searching for anatomical-pathological causes of disorders such as schizophrenia, mania, and what was then known as "hysteria" (conditions the pathological origins of which we have yet to identify to this day). Meanwhile, doctors were assuming that other mental diseases (which we now know are caused by pathological processes), such as the "general paresis of the insane" (i.e., paralytic dementia) that appears in late-stage syphilis, were actually primary mental disorders. Sigmund Freud, for example, started out as a neuropathologist looking for the organic brain lesions of schizophrenia, which neither he nor anyone else yet has found. He gave up in frustration to become one of the founders of psychiatry in order to study the nonphysical dimensions of mental illness.

Likewise, the eminent French neurologist Jean Martin Charcot thought that the hypnotic state was a pathological condition akin to hysteria. (His observations, in turn, of tertiary syphilis patients with "general paresis of the insane" who were stumbling around on damaged but painless leg joints led to the pathognomonic attribution of "Charcot joint.") Sigmund Freud, in turn, later retracing Mesmer's journey from Austria to France, met with Charcot at the Hospital Salpetrière in Paris and became fascinated with hypnosis as a tool to explore the subconscious mind in the diagnosis and treatment of neuroses. Later, however, Freud abandoned the technique, striking a blow to its credibility and role in psychiatry and psychology in the succeeding years.[6]

Interest in hypnosis in the medical community again waned. However, later, amid the dislocation, suffering, and trauma of World War II and subsequent wars of the midtwentieth century, hypnosis was again shown to be effective in the treatment of post-traumatic stress disorder (PTSD) and for pain relief.[7] Hypnosis eventually found its way back into mainstream medical practice with an endorsement by the British Medical Association in 1955 and by the American Medical Association and Canadian Medical Association in 1958. Since then, interest in hypnosis has grown, and the practice has found numerous clinical applications. As well, there has lately been a steady stream of clinical research, putting hypnosis on a solid scientific footing.

WHAT IS HYPNOSIS?

Hypnotism consists of two basic components: (1) the use of a technique to induce a state of consciousness that allows greater access to the deeper parts of the mind; and (2) a method for communicating with those deeper parts of the mind. This kind of communication involves making suggestions to ("the power of suggestion") and evoking images in the inner depths of the mind. The hypnotist suggests items or behaviors that you may desire for your betterment. But first, you must be placed in a state of hypnosis.

Several different techniques are used to induce the necessary state of consciousness, and some may be quite similar to some of the more common relaxation techniques and to meditation. Physiologically, in terms of its effects, hypnosis resembles other forms of deep relaxation discussed in this book. It decreases nervous-system activity, decreases oxygen consumption, and lowers blood pressure and heart rate. It can also increase or decrease certain types of brain-wave activity. Hypnotherapy's effectiveness lies in the complex connections between the mind and the body. It is now understood that illness and pain affect your emotional state, and conversely, that your emotional state affects your physical state. For example, stress, an emotional reaction, can make pain or heart disease worse. And heart disease, a physical condition, can cause depression as well as physical pain.

Hypnosis carries this connection another logical step by using the power of the mind to bring about changes in the body. No one is quite sure how hypnosis works, but with more sophisticated brain-imaging techniques, scientists are beginning to be able see where and how the brain "thinks" in various emotional-mental states of hypnosis, meditation, prayer, and so on.

Like many other functions of the human brain, the precise physiological mechanisms of hypnosis still aren't fully understood. On a superficial level, people under hypnosis appear to be asleep, but their EEG brain-wave patterns resemble wakefulness.[8] The difference between normal wakefulness and the hypnotic state appears to reside in the locations where the brain-wave activity occurs. Neurological studies of hypnotized people using EEGs have shown a shift of brain-wave activity to different regions of the brain. However, imagining colors while hypnotized results in measurable increases in blood flow to the visual cortex, the area of the brain that is normally stimulated during actual sight.[9]

HOW IT WORKS

You've no doubt seen hypnosis depicted in the movies, where the hypnotist swings a pocket watch in front of a person's face as he says, "You're getting sleepy . . ." But I have never seen this technique used in real life (nor do you see a lot of pocket watches around anymore). That said, there is no uniform method for inducing hypnosis. However, there are three common features in most applications of clinical hypnosis: (1) absorption in the words or images presented by the hypnotherapist; (2) dissociation from your ordinary critical faculties; and (3) responsiveness to the suggestions presented by the hypnotherapist ("the power of suggestion").

A hypnotherapist either leads the person through relaxation, mental imagery, and suggestions or teaches the person to perform the techniques him- or herself. Many hypnotherapists provide guided audiotapes for their patients so that they can practice the therapy at home on their own. The images presented in such recordings are specifically tailored to the particular person's unique needs and may use one or all of the five (or six, if you include extrasensory perception) senses.

A hypnosis session usually incorporates five steps or phases:

1. **Preparation:** You are placed in a comfortable, secure environment, usually sitting in a quiet room. Distractions and interruptions are minimized.
2. **Induction:** You are guided to a state of relaxation by deep breathing, progressive muscle relaxation, and/or the use of imagery.
3. **Deepening:** In this phase, the hypnotic state is deepened through repetition and reinforcement. Conscious thinking is minimized.

4. **Purpose:** This phase is where the specific goal of the hypnosis is addressed. Hypnotic suggestions are given to modify perceptions or behavior. For example, in the case of pain management, you may be asked to transform the perception of pain to a numbness or tingling sensation.

5. **Awakening:** In this final phase, you're gradually brought out of the hypnotic state. During this stage, the therapeutic suggestions presented during step 4 are repeated and reinforced as the level of hypnosis lightens. Then the hypnotherapist offers some final suggestions before you emerge into normal consciousness, typically refreshed and relaxed.

Usually, a hypnosis session produces immediate positive results. People also report a sense of well-being and calm, although they're often uncertain about how deeply they were "under." They often comment on how they were completely aware of what was going on, but with a curious unconcern about their surroundings. Subsequent sessions usually produce deeper levels of hypnosis, since patients are usually less apprehensive about the technique and feel safer at this point.

A typical hypnosis session takes between thirty minutes and an hour, and there are no studies or guidelines about the optimal frequency of sessions. Weekly sessions are probably realistic for most people, and they are encouraged to practice self-hypnosis between sessions. The self-hypnosis method, while not quite as effective as guided therapy with a skilled hypnotherapist, requires you to use your own skills in achieving a hypnotic state by applying the breathing techniques and imagery that you learn during your regular sessions with the therapist.

What Is It Like to Be Hypnotized?

By most accounts, hypnosis is characterized by increased mental focus and concentration, an indifference to the external environment, and heightened receptiveness or susceptibility to suggestion. The facilitation of this "suggestibility" appears to come from an inclination by the hypnotized person to suspend the censoring of received information (i.e., in the higher centers of the cortex of the brain). Most people describe a pleasantly altered state of consciousness (but not sleep), an air of calmness, and a general feeling of well-being while under hypnosis. When properly performed, hypnosis is almost always accompanied by reduced feelings of anxiety and stress. It has been likened to a state of "highly focused attention with a constriction in peripheral awareness."[10]

There is controversy about whether a deep level of hypnosis is required to achieve therapeutic effects. Most recent studies suggest that deep hypnosis is not necessary, and a large percentage of people can benefit from even light levels of hypnosis, while a smaller percentage will be able to achieve complete hypnotic anesthesia.

Hypnotic Susceptibility

It is widely acknowledged that there is considerable variability in individual susceptibility to hypnosis ("hypnotizability"). Most people can be hypnotized to some degree, while perhaps 10 percent cannot be hypnotized at all, and another 10 percent are particularly susceptible.[11] Women are more hypnotizable than men; children are more receptive than adults.

A pioneer of unraveling the myths and mysteries of hypnotism, psychiatrist Herbert Spiegel developed a hypnotic susceptibility scale, known as the Hypnotic Induction Profile or the eye roll test, to provide a biostatistical basis for evaluating receptivity to hypnosis without implying any particular underlying mechanism of action. This approach could in turn provide a basis for the improved, individualized application of other CAM medical modalities and mind-body therapies, in addition to hypnosis, when the mechanism of action is controversial or obscure or remains "foreign" in the view of the contemporary biomedical paradigm.

THE PROVEN EFFECTIVENESS OF HYPNOSIS

The effectiveness of hypnosis has been shown by much more than anecdotal accounts, though there are many of them. Numerous controlled studies on the benefits of hypnotherapy for a wide variety of medical conditions have been published over the years, with a particular emphasis on its value in pain management. A 1999 study at the Mount Sinai Medical School set out to organize and tabulate the extant medical literature on this subject. The field to that point had been in a state of disarray, with numerous anecdotal and uncontrolled reports that had left the medical community uncertain as to the clinical benefits of hypnosis. This study undertook a meta-analysis of nearly twenty previously published trials involving almost a thousand patients. The studies included both clinical patients as well as experimental pain groups with healthy volunteers. Participants included those with pain due to burn injuries, cancer, headaches, coronary disease, and invasive radiologic procedures as well as healthy people given pain under experimental conditions. The results of this meta-analysis revealed significant benefits of hypnotic interventions in the treatment of pain. Effects were more pronounced in highly hypnotizable subjects (about 10 percent). However, those with midrange susceptibility to hypnosis who comprised the largest group in terms of hypnotic susceptibility (about 80 percent) also got significant pain relief from hypnosis intervention.[12] This observation suggests that a deep level of hypnosis is not required to achieve clinical benefits. Moreover, the technique has little downside risk.

Anxiety and Phobias

A 2011 review by the University of Maryland Medical Center shows that hypnosis may help the functioning of the body's immune system and also may provide the kind of relaxation benefits found with other mind-body practices that are effective in easing stress and anxiety.[13]

Hypnosis can be used to establish a new pattern of reacting to stimuli and to reset emotional boundaries around anxiety-producing thoughts and around specific anxiety-causing activities such as stage fright, fear of flying, and other phobias. Typically, the hypnotherapist helps you undo a conditioned physiological response, such as hyperventilation or nausea. This method can also be used to help calm athletes who are preparing to compete. Hypnotherapy can be used to quell almost any fear, whether associated with testing, public speaking, or social interactions.

Dental Pain

Some people have learned to tolerate pain associated with dental work (e.g., drilling, extraction, periodontal surgery) using hypnosis as the sole anesthesia. Even when an anesthetic is used, hypnotherapy can be employed as an adjunct therapy to reduce fear and anxiety, control bleeding and salivation, and lessen postoperative discomfort. Used with children, hypnotherapy can decrease the chances of later developing dental phobias.

A 2000 randomized study involved sixty dental patients scheduled for third molar extraction. The hypnotherapy group received an audiotape incorporating hypnotic induction and suggestions designed to alleviate pain and enhance healing. The treatment group listened to the tape daily in the week preceding oral surgery. Patients receiving hypnotherapy reported less anxiety before their scheduled procedure, although there was no decrease in the consumption of analgesics during the procedure, and so the benefit of the intervention was unclear.[14] Other study groups, however, have discerned greater benefit from hypnosis in dental surgery patients, including a diminished requirement for postoperative analgesics.[15]

Diabetes

A 2011 study showed significant blood sugar–lowering benefits in patients with type 2 diabetes who used hypnosis along with acupressure.[16] Controlling blood sugar in people with diabetes helps prevent the development of painful complications, such as peripheral neuropathy and diabetic pain.

Headache and Chronic Pain

Many controlled studies have demonstrated that hypnosis is an effective way to reduce migraine headache attacks in children and teenagers. In one experiment, thirty schoolchildren were randomly assigned either a placebo, the drug propranolol (a blood pressure–lowering agent), or self-hypnosis. Only the children who used the self-hypnosis techniques had a significant decrease in the severity and frequency of headaches.[17] A 1989 study of chronically ill patients with pain reported an over 100 percent improvement in pain tolerance among highly hypnotizable subjects compared to a control group that did not receive hypnosis.[18]

Irritable Bowel Syndrome

Two studies show impressive benefits of hypnotherapy for people with irritable bowel syndrome. In one, 40 percent of patients in the hypnosis group experienced significant relief, compared to just 12 percent in the control group.[19] In the other study, 85 percent of IBS patients who used hypnosis reported that they still felt the benefits seven years later.[20]

Labor and Childbirth

A noninvasive method to assist in managing childbirth pain is of great importance to obstetric anesthesia practitioners, particularly when epidural anesthesia is impractical or contraindicated. Hypnosis has been used effectively for over a century in the management of childbirth pain,[21] as attested to by a number of recent reports. Women who have used hypnosis before delivery tend to have a shorter labor and more comfortable deliveries than other women. There are even reports of Cesarean sections performed with hypnosis as the sole anesthesia. Women are taught to take advantage of their body's natural anesthetic abilities to make childbirth a less painful, more positive experience.

A 2003 meta-analysis assessed the role of hypnosis in the pain of childbirth and revealed significant benefits. Parturient women who received hypnosis rated their labor pain less severe than controls and required less pharmacological analgesia during labor.[22]

A 2001 study involved a randomized, controlled trial on obstetrical hypnosis in forty-two teenaged mothers-to-be. The young women received a four-session sequence of hypnotic focused relaxation and imagery. Suggestions were directed at participants' ability to manage stress and discomfort. Results showed that those who underwent hypnotherapy had a significantly shorter length of stay in the hospital and fewer complications, and they required less conventional anesthesia during labor and postpartum.[23] It is thought that Lamaze and other popular breathing techniques used during labor and delivery may work by inducing a hypnotic state.

Surgical Pain

Researchers at Virginia Polytechnic Institute found that during a hypnotic state aimed at bringing about pain control, the prefrontal cortex of the brain directed other areas of the brain to reduce or eliminate their awareness of pain.[24] A technique used for surgery in people with little or no tolerance for pharmaceutical anesthesia, a condition called "spinal anesthesia illusion," was developed by Philip Ament, a Buffalo, New York, dentist and psychologist. In this method a deep state of relaxation is induced by having the person count mentally while focusing on a specific image. For the counting intervention, the person is given the suggestion that he or she will feel a growing numbness begin to spread from the navel to the toes while counting higher and higher. Once the person feels numb, the surgery can proceed. After the surgery the therapist gives the person suggestions that lead to the gradual return of normal sensations.[25]

Another meta-analysis that examined the use of hypnosis for general surgical patients involved twenty separate studies and over 1,600 patients. Hypnosis was typically administered in the form of a relaxing induction phase, followed by suggestions aimed at modifying postoperative side effects such as pain, nausea, or distress. Most of the interventions consisted of live sessions administered by a health care professional, while the remainder utilized audiotapes. Results showed broad benefits from hypnosis for a number of clinical outcomes. Nearly 90 percent of patients in the hypnosis groups benefited in comparison to patients receiving standard care. Positive effects included improved levels of anxiety and depression, pain, pain medication use, and physiological indicators such as blood pressure, heart rate, and catecholamine levels. The benefits were similar among both live and audiotape patient groups.[26]

Tinnitus

A 2012 study showed that hypnosis can help alleviate the maddening ringing, buzzing, and hissing in the ears associated with tinnitus.[27]

Tinnitus can be very difficult, leading to anxiety and depression, and it can even be experienced as painful. How hypnosis is able to alleviate tinnitus remains a mystery.

BOUNDARY TYPES: WHO BENEFITS AND WHY

Hypnosis is ideal for thin boundary types. One important way of characterizing a distinctly thin boundary person is that he or she is open to experiences. It makes sense, therefore, that studies have found a correlation between thin boundaries and hypnotic susceptibility. As people on the thin side of the boundary spectrum are better able to identify their feelings than are people on the thick side, they typically respond well to imagery-based approaches such as hypnosis and guided imagery.

FINDING A PRACTITIONER

Hypnotherapy is generally provided by a licensed mental-health practitioner such as a psychiatrist or psychologist or, for dental work, by a dentist who is trained in the clinical practice of hypnosis. A state of trust and confidence should exist between the hypnotherapist and the subject. The patient often requires reassurance, especially at the first session, that there will be no loss of control or inappropriate suggestions. Good practitioners will ease your mind of these worries and allow you to relax—which is, after all, an essential part of any effective mind-body approach, including hypnotherapy.

Getting a personal referral—asking someone you trust who has used hypnotherapy—is always a good way to get leads on qualified professionals. You can also ask for a professional referral from your physician, chiropractor, psychologist, dentist, or other medical professional. They may be working with some knowledge of your medical history that may aid them in recommending a hypnotherapist who specializes in your condition. As well, check with your health insurance to see if your plan covers mental health; if so, you can ask for physicians or other medical personnel in your network who practice hypnosis.

Choosing the right hypnotherapist can be tricky. There are a lot of unaccredited programs that graduate people without the right amount of training. That said, there are also many helpful, professional, well-trained hypnotherapists. It's important to do some solid research before choosing the right hypnotherapist for you. The American Society of Clinical Hypnosis (www.asch.net) is one resource that can help you locate a qualified medical hypnotherapist in your area. The National Board for Certified Clinical Hypnotherapists (www.natboard.com) is another resource geared toward helping people find qualified, board-certified hypnotherapists in their area.

6

Meditation and Yoga

The origins of meditation and yoga are ancient, but the actual science behind their physiological effects is fairly new, as these disciplines have attracted attention from modern Western medicine only in recent years. The Cartesian split between the mind and the body in the early seventeenth century resulted in science emphasizing the body, and Western medicine followed suit, going in the "scientific" direction of studying only the material aspects of the human body. But perceiving the reality of the mind and the body means understanding that the two are not separate; they are interdependent. And meditation and yoga can realign the mind-body to create more harmonious interactions.

MEDITATION

Similar to the word *medicine, meditation* suggests something to do with healing. Physicist David Bohm, in his 1980 book *Wholeness and Implicate Order,* looked at wholeness as a property of the physical, material world. Bohm points out that the Latin root word for medicine and meditation means "to cure," but that its deeper meaning is "to measure."[1] But what does medicine or meditation have to do with measuring? The ancient Greeks said, "Man is the measure of all things." Jon Kabat-Zinn is professor of medicine emeritus and creator of the Center for Mindfulness in Medicine, Health Care, and Society at the University of Massachusetts Medical School. He says, "It has to do with the platonic notion that every shape, every being, every thing has its right inward measure. In other words, a tree has its own quality of wholeness that gives it particular properties. A human being has an individual right inward measure, when everything is balanced and physiologically homeostatic—that's the totality of the individual at that point in time."[2]

Medicine can be seen as the science and art of restoring right inward measure when it is thrown off balance. From the meditative perspective and from the perspective of mind-body medicine, as well as in traditional forms of medicine such as ayurveda and Chinese medicine, health does not have a finite or static destination; it is a dynamic energy flow that changes over a lifetime, with influences toward health and illness coexisting.

Some meditative practices have come to the West from traditional Asian spiritual practices, particularly those of India, China, and Japan. Others can be traced to other ancient cultures, as well as to the strong early American tradition of deliberate, mindful experience of humans in nature.[3] Many Western meditators practice a contemplative, mindful form of meditation as well as other active forms of meditation such as the Chinese martial arts, t'ai chi, the Japanese martial art aikido, and the walking meditations of Zen Buddhism. Yoga also has a devotional, spiritual, meditative aspect to accompany its active aspects. This is the case, for example, for hatha yoga, the form of yoga that emphasizes asanas (yoga positions) and is so popular in the West today; it includes a meditation practice.

Until relatively recently, the primary purpose of meditation has been religious or spiritual in nature. During the past twenty years, however, meditation has been proved to be a healthful means of reducing stress in both mind and body. Many studies have found that various practices of meditation appear to produce physical and psychological changes. Meditation is self-directed and results in relaxing and calming the mind and body. Methods of meditation include focusing on a single thought or word for a specific time. Some forms of meditation focus on a physical experience, such as the breath, or a specific sound or mantra. All forms of meditation have the common objective of stilling the restlessness of the mind so that the focus can be directed inward.

As a health practice, meditation is used to calm the mental activity created by endless, restless thoughts and stressful ways of reacting to our circumstances and environment. As long as accumulated impressions linger in the inner recesses of the mind, nagging for attention—the extent to which we believe relates to your emotional boundary type as delineated in chapter 1—it remains difficult to experience an inner state of peace and calm and an outward state of health and well-being. Fast-paced Western society, filled with external stimuli, has conditioned us to push our minds and bodies to the point of exhaustion, often to the detriment of our own well-being. To be still, to experience the peace and contentment that lies within, we must free ourselves from this external grasping at material reality. Meditation is the process of calming and releasing these distractions from the mind for the purpose of opening up and awakening to our true inner nature.

Mindfulness Meditation

The mindfulness movement in the West was made popular by Jon Kabat-Zinn, PhD, known for his work using mindfulness meditation to help medical patients with chronic pain and stress-related disorders. As with other mind-body therapies, mindfulness meditation can induce deep states of relaxation, can at times improve physical symptoms directly, and can help people lead fuller, more satisfying lives.

While forms of meditation such as Transcendental Meditation (TM) involve focusing on a sound, phrase, or prayer to minimize or eliminate the distraction of the restless mind, the practice of mindfulness does just the opposite. In mindfulness meditation, "distractions" emanating from the outside environment are not ignored but focused on. This form of meditation practice can actually be traced to Buddhist traditions that are about 2,500 years old. The method of mindfulness was developed as a means of cultivating greater awareness and wisdom, with the aim of helping people live each moment of their lives as fully as possible. *New World Mindfulness,* which Micozzi coauthored with Don McCown, points out that there is a distinctive Western and American tradition of mindful contemplation and thought that extends back to the eighteenth century, to the founding fathers John Adams and Thomas Jefferson, and to the leading American philosophers of the nineteenth century, Ralph Waldo Emerson and Henry David Thoreau.[4]

Mindfulness is about more than just feeling relaxed and stress-free; its true aim is to nurture an inner balance that allows a person to face life situations with greater clarity, stability, and understanding and to respond more effectively from that sense of clarity. An integral part of mindfulness practice is to accept and welcome stress, pain, anger, frustration, disappointment, and insecurity when any of those feelings or others are present. Kabat-Zinn believes that acknowledgment is paramount; whether pleasant or unpleasant, admission is the first step toward transforming that reality.

Kabat-Zinn founded the Center for Mindfulness at the University of Massachusetts Medical Center as an outgrowth of his clinical practice. Since the center's founding, more than ten thousand people have gone through its mindfulness meditation programs, almost all of them referred by their physicians. The Center for Mindfulness has published dozens of research studies on mindfulness-based stress reduction. Unlike standard medical and psychological approaches, the center does not categorize and treat people differently based on their illness; the eight-week courses taught there offer the same training program in mindfulness and stress reduction to everyone. The emphasis is on what's "right" with people rather than what's "wrong" with them, focusing on mobilizing their inner strengths and changing their behaviors in new and innovative ways. Facilitators maintain that their programs are not held out as some kind of magical cure-all after other approaches have failed; rather, they provide a sensible and straightforward way for people to experience and understand the mind-body connection firsthand, using that knowledge to better cope with whatever physical problem they are dealing with.

Mindfulness Training

In the practice of mindfulness, the person begins by using directed attention in the moment to cultivate calmness and stability. When thoughts and feelings arise, it is important not to ignore them, suppress them, or analyze or judge them by their content; rather, the thoughts are observed intentionally and nonjudgmentally, moment by moment, as events in a field of awareness.

This inclusive noting of thoughts that come and go in the mind can lead to a detachment from them, allowing a deeper perspective about the stresses of life to emerge. By observing the thoughts from this more distant vantage point, one gains a new frame of reference. In this way, valuable insights can be allowed to surface. The key to mindfulness practice is not the particular topic of attention but the quality of awareness brought into each moment. Observing the thought processes without intellectualizing them and without judgment creates greater clarity. The goal of mindfulness practice is to become more aware, more in touch with life and its happenings at the time they are actually happening—now, in the present moment. Acceptance does not mean passivity or resignation. Accepting what each moment offers provides the opportunity to experience life more completely. In this manner, any situation can be handled with greater confidence and clarity.

One way to envision how mindfulness works is by thinking of the mind as the surface of a lake or ocean. Many people think the goal of meditation is to stop the waves so that the water will be flat, peaceful, and tranquil. The spirit of mindfulness practice is to experience the wetness, the waves, and the ripples on the surface of the water, but in a somewhat detached way.

The Proven Effectiveness of Mindfulness Practice

The consistent practice of mindfulness meditation has been shown to decrease the subjective experience of pain and stress in a variety of research settings. In one study, a 65 percent improvement in pain symptoms and an approximate 60 percent improvement in sleep and fatigue levels occurred after mindfulness meditation in seventy-seven people suffering from fibromyalgia.[5]

Another study used electroencephalographic (EEG) recordings to differentiate between two types of meditation, concentration and mindfulness, and a normal relaxation situation as a control. Results showed significant differences between readings at numerous cortical sites, suggesting that concentration and mindfulness meditations may be unique forms of consciousness and not merely set degrees of a state of relaxation.[6]

In a study using mindfulness of movement as a coping strategy for multiple sclerosis, participants attended six one-on-one sessions of mindfulness training; results of the training revealed significant improvements in the people involved.[7]

Eighty cancer patients were followed for six months after attending a mindfulness meditation group for an hour and a half each week for seven weeks. They were also asked to practice meditation at home on a daily basis. Results showed significantly lower mood disturbances and fewer symptoms of stress at the six-month follow-up for both male and female participants. The greatest improvement occurred on the subscales that measured depression, anxiety, and anger.[8]

Nurses are often known to make mindfulness practice part of their continuing education. They find that this technique often prevents compassion fatigue and burnout, enhances health, and increases awareness of holism within the self.

Transcendental Meditation

In 1955, Maharishi Mahesh Yogi introduced the Transcendental Meditation (TM) technique and the TM movement in India as a simple and practical form of meditation for householders and busy working people, as opposed to the more esoteric meditation traditions practiced by Indian yogis and spiritual masters that had prevailed for centuries. He initiated thousands of people in this technique and developed a teacher-training program. Then the Maharishi inaugurated a series of world tours to introduce TM to the West.

TM has its origins in ancient Vedic philosophy. The Maharishi eliminated the esoteric yogic elements that he considered unnecessary or impractical in a contemporary setting. Omitting difficult physical postures and exercises, his reformed (watered-down) version of this form of meditation became more readily accepted and practiced by Westerners. On the Maharishi's first visit to America in 1959, a San Francisco newspaper heralded TM as a "non-medicinal tranquilizer" and praised it as a promising cure for insomnia.[9] TM soon began to ride a crest of popularity, with almost half a million Americans learning the technique by 1975. It was embraced by many celebrities of the day, most famously the Beatles (before their mindful breakup). It is believed that about two million people currently practice TM in the United States, and millions more worldwide.

How Is It Done?

TM is relatively simple to learn. In the basic training you are given a mantra (a special word or sound) to repeat silently over and over again, with eyes closed, while sitting in a comfortable position. The purpose of repeating the mantra is to prevent distracting thoughts from entering your mind. You are instructed to be passive, and if thoughts other than the mantra come to mind, you note them and return your attention to the mantra. TM is generally practiced in the morning and in the evening for approximately fifteen to twenty minutes.

The Proven Effectiveness of TM

In 1968, mind-body medicine pioneer Herbert Benson was asked by the Maharishi International University in Fairfield, Iowa, to test TM practitioners on their ability to lower their own blood pressure. Benson initially refused to participate but was later persuaded to do so. His studies and other subsequent research showed that TM was associated with reduced health care costs, increased longevity, and better quality of life. Benson also found reduced anxiety, lowered blood pressure, and reduced serum cholesterol levels.[10] TM has also been used as a viable treatment of post-traumatic stress disorder in Vietnam War veterans and for reduction of chronic pain.[11]

YOGA

The origins of yoga date back to ancient times, perhaps as early as five thousand years ago. The word *yoga* comes from the Sanskrit word *yug*, meaning "to join" or "to yoke." It connotes the joining of the lower human nature to the higher. The Puranic Age was from 500 to

1300 CE. The Puranas, a vast genre of Indian literature about a wide range of topics, including philosophical, mythological, and ritual knowledge, were created during this time. The Sectarian Age, from 1300 to 1700 CE, included the bhakti movement, the theistic devotional trend that emerged in medieval Hinduism. The Modern Age began round 1700 CE, during which time there was a growing political presence of European nations in India. At about this time, the exchange and spread of Hindu wisdom and traditions to the West, which some time later included hatha yoga, occurred. This in fact influenced "orientalists" and early practitioners of meditation (or what they called "contemplation") in Europe and America, including the aforementioned Adams, Jefferson, Emerson, Thoreau, and others.

Ancient Vedic texts describe various types of yogic practices. These include bhakti yoga (which emphasizes spirituality and devotion), jnana yoga (which emphasizes attainment of wisdom), karma yoga (which emphasizes offering services without selfish motive), raja yoga (which emphasizes mastering the mind by focused concentration), dhyana yoga (which emphasizes meditation), mantra yoga (which emphasizes repetition of sacred recitations), and hatha yoga (which emphasizes the psychophysical energies of the body).

Hatha yoga, as we now know it, is a relatively recent development compared to other forms of yoga and is the most well-known and popular form of yoga here in the United States. It has three essential components: (1) *asanas,* physical exercises and postures; (2) *pranayama,* breathing techniques; and (3) meditation or concentration and mindfulness practice. It is claimed that the practice of hatha yoga allows a person to alter his or her mental and bodily responses, many typically thought to be beyond one's control. It facilitates an elevation of self-awareness and can ultimately lead to attaining a state of enlightenment. From a health standpoint, yoga promotes physical, mental, social, and spiritual well-being. Hatha yoga focuses on developing the body's physical potential to prepare for self-transcendence. As such, it can be considered a system to purify the body. It is the most explicitly physical form, and for this reason, not surprisingly, it is the branch of yoga most widely recognized in the West. Unfortunately, some Western practitioners of hatha yoga do not always adhere to the ethical principles or spiritual goals of this form of yoga, and in some cases it is used solely for the purpose of physical fitness or as a social interaction.

However, there are other ancient forms of yoga that deserve mention. Raja yoga is a branch of yoga involving adherence to the eightfold path described by Indian sage Patañjali in the Yoga Sutras, with the main practice being meditation. *Raja* means "royal." This word may reflect the belief that raja yoga is superior to hatha yoga because traditionally it called for a monastic life and required years of practice and meditation to master. It is also possible that this path is known by this name because it was practiced by Indian kings.[12]

Bhakti means "devotion," and bhakti yoga is the path of devotion to a deity or a guru as a representative of the deity, and commitment to the love of the divine as the Beloved.[13] This devotion expresses itself in worship in song, ritual, or meditation. The final moment of transcendence is when the practitioner merges with the Beloved in a state of pure love.

Jnana (*gyana*) means "knowledge" or "wisdom," and it is the path associated with discerning what is real without the subconscious clouding the clarity.[14] This path involves deep exploration, contemplation, and study to achieve direct knowledge of the divine and to eliminate what is illusion.

Karma yoga is the yoga of action and service. It is based on the teachings of the Bhagavad Gita that describe an inner attitude to the actions of daily living. The action is selfless activity that transcends the ego and is a means to merging with the divine.[15]

Styles of Yoga

The physical aspects of yoga were, for most of yoga's long history, esoteric techniques practiced only by a few yogis in secret. Krishnamacharya (1888–1989), "the Father of Modern Yoga," was an Indian yoga teacher and ayurvedic healer who is credited with the development of modern hatha yoga as we know it today, as a means to improve physical health and well-being. Krishnamacharya's students included most of yoga's most renowned twentieth-century healers, each of whom developed unique schools or styles of yoga that have become the most well-regarded styles of yoga in the United States today: T. K. V. Desikachar, Indra Devi, B. K. S. Iyengar, K. Pattabhi Jois, and A. G. Mohan.

T. K. V. Desikachar (1938–2016), the son of Krishnamacharya, went on to develop Viniyoga, "a highly individualized approach to yoga that tailors the practice to each student's specific physical condition, emotional state, age, cultural background, and interests."[16] Classes include instruction in asana, pranayama, meditation, yoga philosophy, and Vedic chanting. Desikachar trained many teachers in the United States and at his center in India, which has pioneered research into the impact of yoga on people suffering from schizophrenia, diabetes, asthma, and depression. "Yoga is basically a program for the spine at every level—physical, respiratory, mental, and spiritual," says Desikachar.[17]

Colorful, Russian-born Indra Devi (1899–2002), "the First Lady of Yoga," became an influential yoga teacher in the West after coming to the United States in 1947 and opening a yoga studio in Hollywood that attracted celebrities, and thereafter a number of adherents. Devi was among the first in the West to write books on yoga, and her books influenced many modern Western teachers today.[18] Her method stresses the correct use of the breath, and slow-paced classes often include a pause in savasana (corpse pose) after every nonresting pose in order to become aware of each asana's effects.

B. K. S. Iyengar (1918–2014) was the founder of the style known as Iyengar yoga, which now has several established teacher-training and practice centers in the United States that have trained thousands of Iyengar yoga teachers. Iyengar yoga emphasizes building physical strength matched with flexibility. Iyengar believed in adapting the pose to the individual, and to accomplish this his style of yoga uses a number of props to help students gain correct physical alignment.

K. Pattabhi Jois (1915–2009) was the innovator behind a gymnastic style of yoga known as Ashtanga. In a typical Ashtanga class the student learns a series of linked poses, known as *vinyasa,* combined with yogic breathing. In a typical Ashtanga class the student proceeds through each of the linked poses at his or her own pace, with the teacher available to oversee and assist as necessary. Ashtanga classes are fast-moving and athletic.

A. G. Mohan (b. 1945) developed a system of yoga called Svastha, a Sanskrit word that means "to stay in one's own abode," referring to the state of complete health and balance. His method incorporates asana, pranayama, and traditional ayurveda (Mohan is also an ayurvedic healer). Svastha yoga emphasizes yogic mindfulness, including minding your body, breath, mind, senses, speech, and food, to attain a calm, clear, light, balanced mode of mind, a state called *sattva* in Sanskrit.

In addition to these styles of yoga, what has come to be known in the twentieth century as Kundalini yoga is a synthesis of many traditions that includes haṭha yoga postures, along with kriya yoga (consisting of self-discipline, self-study, and devotion to God), tantric visualization, and meditation techniques. The goal of Kundalini yoga is to awaken the person's kundalini energy, the spiritual energy or life force located at the base of the spine, conceptualized as a coiled-up serpent. The practice of Kundalini yoga is supposed to arouse the sleeping kundalini power from its coiled base through the six chakras (or energy centers of the body) so that it penetrates the seventh chakra, or crown, to bring about an awakened or enlightened state.

Bikram yoga is a form hatha yoga found in many cities in the United States. It consists of a set series of twenty-seven copyrighted postures and breathing, developed by the controversial yoga figure Bikram Choudhury. The exercises are done in a room that is heated to 105 degrees Fahrenheit. Benefits include protecting the muscles and allowing for deeper stretching, opening the pores to release toxins, better blood circulation, improved strength, and improved heart rate for a better cardiovascular workout. However, as the heat and postures of Bikram are fairly intense, it may not be the most compatible style for people with chronic pain.

How Is It Done?

A hatha yoga session in a class or group setting (yoga can also be practiced individually at home) varies widely in content and duration based on the teacher, the group being taught, and especially the school or system of yoga being taught, as mentioned above. While it's impossible to describe the average yoga session, more than likely a typical class will be anywhere from forty-five minutes to an hour and a half. Most classes begin with breathing exercises that require long, deep nostril breathing that assists in quieting the mind. The next phase involves gentle exercises and postural movements to facilitate strength and flexibility of the joints and muscles, usually followed by somewhat more difficult postures, or asanas. A final resting period, typically in the recumbent corpse pose (savasana), is often followed by chanting the sacred syllable *Om* while seated in a prayerful position at the conclusion of the class. However, this description does not necessarily fit every style of yoga, and some styles are far more athletic and demanding while others are more focused on the meditative aspects of yoga, as originally intended.

Many difficult and cumbersome postures and athletic styles of yoga are contraindicated in certain musculoskeletal and other chronic pain conditions or as dictated by age and physical fitness. Physical damage to muscles, ligaments, and joints can occur if the yoga practitioner is attempting to do something that is beyond his or her skill level. Those with balance problems and severe pain should also be cautious of certain styles of yoga. Practitioners who are starting out in yoga are advised to exercise gently and slowly and to not stretch beyond their comfort levels. All asanas should be performed with a certain amount of ease, never forcing the posture.

Yoga practice involves the total body and total mind. It provides a powerful way of controlling physiological processes and also of controlling physiological reactions to psychological events.

Combining Yoga and Nature

Consider doing yoga in the great outdoors! The more often you do it there, the longer you'll want to practice. Yoga practiced outdoors in nature offers a vast array of health benefits. It can help lower the risk of heart disease and reduce stress, anxiety, and depression. In one study, researchers found that men and women significantly reduced their stress when they practiced in a forest compared to indoors.[19] In another study, researchers found that men and women who practiced in parks and forests reduced their stress-induced headaches.[20]

But you don't need to do a yoga workout in nature to gain nature's benefits. Yoga goes beyond the postures on your mat. Just spending ten minutes a day walking in a park can lower your blood pressure, and when done mindfully this can be part of your yoga practice. Spending time out in nature has a meditative, energetic, and even spiritual aspect to it. Very often I think we mistake being active and moving around as being superior to actually slowing down. Being out in nature helps cultivate the nonphysical aspects of yoga, such as appreciating the stillness between movements. Ernest Hemingway wrote, "Never confuse motion with action." It seems that being in perpetual, strenuous motion is not really the best way to achieve good health. We also know it's quite possible and increasingly common to overdo it. This reminds us of our discussion above of the importance of cultivating ease in a yoga practice and avoiding the tendency to use yoga as purely physical fitness. Indeed, extreme exercise takes a toll on the joints and heart muscle in the long term. By comparison, studies show that gentle exercise or movement, including not only yoga but also swimming, walking, or gardening, gives you more benefits from a practical health standpoint than all the obsessive "conditioning" that takes place in a gym.

The Proven Effectiveness of Yoga

Yoga elicits a relaxation response characterized by lower consumption of oxygen, lower heart and respiration rates, and changes in brain activity. Yoga alters various pulmonary, cerebral, mental, and metabolic physiological functions, producing beneficial effects on the central nervous and cardiovascular systems. These beneficial effects include an increase in verbal creativity, reduced visual reaction time and intra-ocular pressure, better breath-holding ability, improved tidal volume (lung volume) and vital capacity (the maximum amount of air a person can expel from the lungs after a maximum inhalation), an improvement in physical fitness, reduction in anxiety, and improved blood sugar levels, particularly among diabetics.[21]

One of the most important changes that take place in the body during meditation and yoga practice is the slowing down of the metabolism, resulting in a sharp reduction in oxygen consumption and carbon dioxide output, by as much as 20 percent.[22] Although blood pressure and heart rate decrease overall, peripheral blood flow increases during meditation; activities of the sympathetic nervous system are reduced, and constriction of the blood vessels is decreased. This peripheral blood flow ensures that oxygen is more efficiently delivered to the muscles and that lactate is more quickly and effectively removed. Reduction of lactate level has a direct effect on reduction of blood pressure and anxiety levels.

The quality of relaxation produced by both yoga and meditation may be deeper than that produced by sleep, allowing recuperation of the body from the damaging effects of overproduction of adrenaline and activity of the sympathetic nervous system. Ideally, proper activation and optimal performance of the brain leads to a life of relaxation, which at the same time, is more efficient and disease-free.

A distinct phase of relaxation, referred to as the "fourth state of consciousness" (the other three being waking, dreaming, and sleeping), has been described in conjunction with yoga practice. This state is characterized by the usual changes seen in deep relaxation, such as reduced cortisol and plasma lactate levels, decreased muscle and red blood cell metabolism, and reduced breath rate. In addition, this fourth state also produces increased alpha brain-wave activity and a distinctive pattern of enhanced cerebral blood flow. The regular practice of yoga has also been shown to have positive effects on mood and emotional well-being, improved muscle strength, and relaxation.[23]

In a general, hatha yoga, including asanas (postures), breath work, and meditation, produces a state of relaxation and improves muscle strength. The relaxation response is associated with a lower level of anxiety and reduced sympathetic drive.

Yoga has been demonstrated to be effective in the management of arthritis, low-back pain, and headaches.[24] The evidence for its ability to improve mood and quality of life in those with chronic illnesses is considerable.[25] Yoga has also been successfully used in the treatment of anxiety, insomnia, and various neurological conditions.[26] Conditions like Alzheimer's disease and other disorders of the brain that affect memory and concentration are on the rise. Researchers at the University of Illinois recently studied 108 inactive people between the ages of fifty-five and seventy-nine. Participants who did yoga three times a week for eight weeks experienced improved memory and mental skills, while those who only did stretching and toning exercises did not receive any cognitive benefits.[27] It appears that engaging in a "mindful" practice like yoga provides more benefits than simple "mindless" exercise.

Research was conducted by Julie Staples, a certified Kundalini yoga teacher who is research director at the Center for Mind-Body Medicine in Washington, D.C., as well as an adjunct assistant professor in the department of physiology and biophysics at Georgetown University School of Medicine. Staples and her associates conducted a study to see how yoga practice affected adults age sixty-five to eighty-five. They looked at three major conditions that impact memory and cognition: poor sleep, pain, and stress. For three months, participants in the study practiced yoga daily at home. The holistic therapy program consisted of postures, breathing exercises, chants, gestures (mudras), conscious intention, relaxation, and diet. Following the study, participants reported significant improvements in sleep quality, pain levels, and energy levels. When asked if they enjoyed participating in the program, 92 percent gave it the two highest ratings, and 100 percent said they would recommend the program to others.[28]

A number of musculoskeletal disorders and common occupational health problems may be managed with yoga, including carpal tunnel syndrome, osteoarthritis, and low-back pain.[29] Preliminary evidence indicates that yoga may also be helpful in disorders of the immune system, such as rheumatoid arthritis and lupus.[30] Constant and repeated cycles of stress can compromise many normal physiological processes and contribute to pain; several controlled trials have shown that yoga reduces stress, anxiety, and depression, all symptoms associated with pain.[31]

Increases in your pulse rate over the long term can have negative effects on the cardiovascular system. Research shows that meditation combined with yoga reduces mild to moderate high blood pressure. Thirty years ago, researchers in Europe studied blood pressure treatment guidelines. They found that half the world's population would be considered at risk for hypertension by the age of twenty-four when using the 120/80 blood-pressure standard considered normal, and 90 percent would be at risk by the age of forty-nine.[32] These numbers account for more than three-quarters of the world's entire adult population—quite a prime market for drug companies.

In a recent clinical trial, University of Pennsylvania researchers studied 120 people, average age fifty, with mild to moderate high blood pressure, the average systolic blood pressure reading being 134 mm Hg. The researchers gave the participants three treatment options: yoga, diet, and yoga and diet combined. They divided the participants into three groups. One group practiced yoga two or three times a week in a studio; the second group began a walking regimen and received nutritional counseling; and the third group practiced yoga plus received dietary counseling.

Findings showed that men and women who practiced yoga reduced their systolic blood pressure by 5 to 6 mg Hg after twelve weeks, in contrast to the non-yoga group, which did not show any significant changes. The lead researcher in this investigation reported, "It's not a huge decrease in blood pressure; it's not a drug effect; but it is significant."[33] Certainly from this study one can conclude that for those experiencing the early signs of high blood pressure (in the mild to moderate range), a lifestyle modification like yoga can potentially help keep you off drugs.

An eight-week study on Bikram yoga conducted at Boise State University found that hot yoga positively affected psychological and physical health in the sample population and gave people the tools to decrease perceived stress, potentially having an effect on chronic stress-related illnesses.[34]

BOUNDARY TYPES: WHO BENEFITS AND WHY

Yoga (especially hatha yoga) may often be well suited to the needs of thick boundary individuals because of the physical, bodily aspects of the practice. Meditation may be especially useful for people with thick boundaries because they typically need to get in better touch with their feelings. By slowing down and focusing in a structured practice of meditation or yoga, those with thick boundaries can better come to perceive what is going on inside them.

Of course, relaxation is a necessary step for almost any mind-body therapy to work for anyone, thick or thin boundary. Meditation and yoga are two avenues to relaxation and therefore everyone on the boundary-type spectrum could potentially benefit from their relaxation effects.

FINDING A TEACHER

Many people learn to teach mindfulness-based meditation nationally and worldwide.* These teachers do not think of themselves as practitioners per se as they believe their students are doing the important work. Teachers typically meet with students in groups of around eight to twelve people for eight weekly meetings. A good resource for finding a mindfulness teacher is through a practitioner of one of the other mind-body techniques addressed in this book. You can also always search online for mindfulness classes and groups in your area.

In yoga, the individual's consciousness is thought to be connected with the physical body at the heart. This consciousness, in an "unenlightened" person, is called "self-contraction." This contraction is felt at the level of the heart as a sense of separation, isolation, loneliness, fear, and uncertainty. At the level of the mind, this contraction manifests itself as doubt. Yoga endeavors to expand this contraction. Unfortunately, in the West, yoga has sometimes been reduced to fitness training bereft of the consciousness and spirit element that can be brought to the heart and mind. Although reductionist yoga practice helps many people maintain and restore physical health, it does not provide the full potential benefits of yoga. Many practitioners of

---

*There have been many books written on teaching mindfulness, including Donald McCown, Diane K. Reibel, and Marc S. Micozzi's *Teaching Mindfulness: A Practical Guide for Clinicians and Educators*, 2nd edition (New York: Springer, 2016).

yoga, particularly in the West, know only this reductionist form of yoga.

Yoga was never intended for quick fixes or as a cheap service to the ego. Promises of enlightenment over a weekend or a week are misconceptions. Like anything in life, the benefits of yoga practice are commensurate with the attention, discipline, and effort put into it. Yoga must be learned from a knowledgeable and experienced teacher. A mature student will have no difficulty in learning from a master in any given field. We must, however, examine our teachers carefully. As proven constantly in our daily experience, neither education nor age is any guarantee of wisdom. The mass media has profitably manipulated public opinion by confusing the guru tradition with the vexing issues of cult leadership and brainwashing. As more flamboyant and questionable gurus are replaced by true teachers and spiritual masters, the maturing of yoga in the West should follow.

That said, there are several ways to find the right yoga teacher for you. You can often find local teachers and schools by searching online. Often you can find a schedule of classes and any other information they have that might be useful to a new student on their website, or you can find contact information to contact the teacher or school directly. Or ask your friends or associates at work to recommend a teacher or yoga studio. Once you've gathered all of your information, talk to someone at each school or studio and speak to the teacher of the class you're interested in—and if you're new to yoga it's best to start out in a beginner's class. Find out something about the school's approach; some classes, like Ashtanga, are notoriously vigorous, while others, like Viniyoga, are much milder.

If you have any physical problems or limitations, briefly describe them to the teacher and see if he or she feels comfortable working with you. You might ask about his or her training, certifications, and teaching experience. If you're able to sample a few different teachers, try one or more classes with each one before settling on someone you know you want to study with.

In starting yoga it is important to *never* perform any position in class that generates "bad" pain, especially in the knees, lower back, and neck. Don't suffer in silence if you're forcing a posture that hurts in a yoga class. Either tell the teacher what you're experiencing and ask for an alternative position, or stop altogether and assume a resting posture until the class is ready to move on. And be sure to provide feedback to the teacher at the end of class so that he or she is aware of any limitations you might have.

7
Spiritual Healing

Throughout the ages, ancient mystical and theological traditions have valued the spiritual qualities of humans over their physical qualities, emphasizing the transcendence of the one over the other. In the background of most mystical traditions is the idea that the body is somehow at odds with the spirit, or, in terms of our book, that the boundary conditions are not "right"; the body does not represent the essence of the spirit and these different domains of existence do not fully overlap. A war wages, and one must fight this war to achieve an enlightened state. Still other theologians postulate that the greatest spiritual achievement of all may lie in the realization that the spiritual and the physical are one, and that perhaps the ultimate spiritual goal is to transcend nothing, but rather to realize this integration and bring into view the oneness of being that always, already, simply exists.

A new quality of spiritual awakening has been emerging worldwide over the past three decades that may be seen to parallel developments in quantum physics. An innovative approach encourages people to develop faith in their own capacity to create their own reality in partnership with the God-force within. In many cultures, both Eastern and Western, prayer-based spiritual healing is an integral part of modern religious practices. The premise of creating our own reality is, in essence, a spiritual one. This concept is sometimes contrary to the dualism of many traditional and fundamentalist religions that see God as an entirely external being or entity. Transcending the boundaries and limitations of specific religions, a personal spiritual practice that honors the relationship between the individual and the God-force as a partnership lies at the heart of this new movement.

When people consider the possibility that they create their own realities, the questions that invariably arise are: (1) through what source? or (2) what is the source of this power of creation that runs through my being? The answers are found not externally, but internally. This internal source seeking to understand our own nature is the study of divinity in action, which each human being possesses.

The blending of spirituality with the tenets of CAM therapies provides us with a means of understanding how we ourselves help contribute to the creation of illness and to our healing. This consideration does not come from a place of self-blame and is not a result of the "will of God"; rather it comes from attempting to understand a spiritual reason underlying suffering in a physical body. The relationship that is cultivated ultimately transcends the value system of punishment versus reward and grows into a relationship based on principles of co-creation and co-responsibility. In this way the journey of healing as well as the journey of life is freed of the burden of feeling victimized by fate, circumstances, or God; we become free to have faith and hope not only in God but in ourselves as well.

USING CONSCIOUSNESS TO CURE

In addition to the recognized psychotherapies of mainstream Western biomedicine, there are various modalities of mind-body medicine such as those described in this book that are widely considered to be effective for overcoming pain and associated mood disorders. However, spiritual healing, an important but perhaps more amorphous modality, is often the least understood and perhaps most controversial approach to relieving pain. It may nevertheless be a powerful source of relief for some people, especially when combined with any of the other modalities mentioned in this book.

The idea that consciousness affects the physical body is a

time-honored and respected concept. The observation that there is a measure of consciousness present throughout the body is reflected in medicine going back more than two thousand years, to Hippocrates. In recent times, beyond understanding that the body and mind are connected through the emotions as a contributing source of illness, there is a renewed acceptance of the idea that the mind can help heal physical ailments. Mental healing, or "mind-cure," is part of a long American tradition of mind over matter that dates back to the early nineteenth century, to Phineus Quimby's New Thought movement and to Mary Baker Eddy's philosophy of Christian Science. The idea that mind (which exists beyond the physical brain) can be projected at a distance and used to influence healing (or, conversely, to project malign influences, or curses) is central to mental healing.

Today we have ample evidence that the anatomy, biochemistry, and physiology of the body effectively make the entire body an organ of consciousness. The ancient Persians expounded on this idea in their traditional Unani medicine, as practiced in Mughal India and in Muslim cultures in South Asia and modern-day central Asia. Unani medicine holds the idea that a person's mind can intervene not just in his or her own body, but also in that of another person located far away, thereby extending the emotional boundaries beyond the personal physical body. The great Muslim physician Avicenna (Abu Ali ibn Sina, 980–1037 AD) postulated that it is the faculty of the imagination (a form of mental imagery) that humans use to make themselves ill or to restore health.*

The attitudes of the ancient Greeks and Persians regarding the interactions between the mind and the body gave rise to concepts of two very different varieties of healing: local and nonlocal. The Greeks believed that the action of the mind on the body was a local event, one taking place in the here and now. The Persians, on the other hand, viewed the mind-body relationship as nonlocal. They held that the mind was not localized or confined to the body, but rather extended

---

*For more on this see Mones Abu-Asab, Hakima Amri, and Marc S. Micozzi's *Avicenna's Medicine: A New Translation of the 11th-Century Canon with Practical Applications for Integrative Health Care* (Rochester Vt.: Healing Arts Press, 2013).

beyond the body. This idea implies that the mind is capable of affecting any physical body, self or nonself, whether local or nonlocal.

The Nonlocality of Consciousness

Modern physicists recognize the concept of nonlocality as an integral part of the quantum physics of fundamental particles, which has lately been extended to the biology of living beings. This is based in part on an idea in physics called Bell's theorem, which distinguishes quantum mechanics from the mechanical model and was introduced in 1964 by the Irish physicist John Stewart Bell. Bell showed that if distant objects have at one time been in contact, a change thereafter in one causes an immediate change in the other, even if they are separated to the opposite ends of the universe. Thus it is important to realize that nonlocality is not just a theory, but that its proof rests on actual experimental observations in physics.

The idea that has prevailed in the mechanical model of mainstream science is that the mind and consciousness are entirely local phenomena, localized to the brain/body and confined to the present moment. From this perspective, nonlocal healing cannot occur in principle because the mind is bound by the here and now. However, research studies conducted on distant mental influence challenge these assumptions. Dozens of experiments conducted over the past three decades suggest that the mind can bring about changes in nonlocal physical bodies, even when shielded from all sensory and electromagnetic influences. This observation suggests that mind and consciousness may not be located at fixed points in space.[1]

Where Is Your Mind?

Some physicists believe that nonlocality applies not just to the domain of electrons and other subatomic particles but also to our familiar world of dense matter. And a growing number of physicists think that nonlocality may also apply to the mind. Physicist Nick Herbert, in his book *Quantum Reality,* states, "Bell's theorem requires our quantum knowledge to be non-local, instantly linked to everything it has previously touched."[2]

For the Western model of medicine, the implications of a nonlocal concept are profound and include the following:

- Nonlocal models of the mind could be helpful in understanding the actual dynamics of the healing process. They may help us understand why in some patients a cure appears suddenly, unexpectedly, or spontaneously, or when a healing appears to be influenced by events occurring nonlocally.
- Nonlocal manifestations of consciousness may complicate traditional experimental designs and require innovative research methods because they suggest that the mental state of the healer may influence the experiment's outcome, even under blinded experimental conditions.[3]
- The concept of nonlocality gives rise to the possibility that consciousness prevails after the death of the body/brain, suggesting that some aspect of the psyche is not bound to specific points in space or time. This idea also allows for the possibility of distant healing exchange.
- The nonlocal model of consciousness implies that at some level of the psyche, no fundamental separation exists between individual minds. Nobel physicist Erwin Schroedinger suggested that at some level and in some sense there may be unity and oneness of all minds.[4] In the nonlocal model, distance is not fundamental but is completely overcome. In other words, because of the unification of consciousness, the healer and the patient are not separated by physical distance.

For thirty years, psychologist Lawrence LeShan investigated the local and nonlocal effects of prayer and healing. He taught mental-spiritual healing techniques to more than four hundred people and ultimately became a healer himself. He maintained that when these techniques were used, spontaneous healing changes that could not have been predicted ahead of time were observed to have occurred in 15 to 20 percent of cases.[5] LeShan found that mental-spiritual healing methods are of the following two main types:

Type 1 (nonlocal). The healer enters a prayerful, altered state of consciousness in which he or she views him- or herself and the patient as a single entity. There is no physical contact or any attempt to offer anything of a physical nature to the person in need, only the desire to connect and unite. Healers of this type emphasize the importance of empathy, love, and caring in this process. When the healing takes place, it does so in the context of unity, compassion, and love. This type of healing is considered a natural process and merely speeds up the normal healing processes.

Type 2 (local). The healer does touch the patient and may imagine some flow of energy through his or her hands to the patient. Feelings of heat are common in both the healer and the patient. In this mode, unlike type 1, the healer holds the intention for healing.

Research about the origins of consciousness and how it relates to the physical brain is practically nonexistent. Although hypotheses purporting to explain consciousness do exist, there is no agreement among researchers as to its nature and whether it is local or nonlocal. While a scientific basis for mental healing is provided by theoretical, fundamental physics and experimentation, there is no single, specific mind-body technique per se in the traditions of these practitioners.

The Healing Power of Positive Emotions

It is not just the mind that can heal; feelings and emotions, very much influenced by the mind, are also involved. Being emotionally touched by, or feeling, the beauty of nature, music, or art is certainly good for the soul, but there is also evidence that these kinds of experiences are good for your physical health too. A new study, one of the first to discover the biochemical mechanisms by which positive emotions can improve health, shows that these emotions may reduce inflammation, a major culprit behind everything from depression to diabetes to heart disease and some cancers.[6] Researchers involved in this investigation conducted two experiments on more than two hundred young adults. Participants reported when they experienced emotions such as amusement, awe, compassion, contentment, joy, love, or pride each day. Then the scientists took samples of each person's cheek and gum tissues and measured the levels of cytokines in those tissues. Cytokines are proinflammatory proteins whose role is to signal the immune system to boost its activity to help fight off an infection, virus, or other trauma. But too many cytokines result in chronic inflammation, which can lead to disorders like arthritis, Alzheimer's, depression, diabetes, and heart disease—not to mention overall poor health. The researchers found that study participants with the highest levels of positive emotions also had the lowest levels of cytokines, as well as another marker of inflammation found in white blood cells.

It appears that positive emotions can help stave off chronic inflammation and a host of chronic diseases, but they may also help with temporary symptoms as well. Elevated cytokines and chronic inflammation in the brain appears to block key hormones and neurotransmitters that influence appetite, memory, mood, and sleep. For instance, it has long been said that people with seasonal allergies are more likely to suffer from depression. Perhaps the effects of cytokines and chronic inflammation play a role in this association. So positive emotions have the potential for some far-reaching health benefits.

The Power of Prayer

The use of prayer in healing may have begun in human prehistory and continues to this day as an underlying tenet in almost all charismatic religions. The records of many of the great religious traditions, including the mystical traditions of Christianity, Taoism, Hinduism, Buddhism, and Islam, all give the strong impression that enlightenment comes when one begins to explore the dynamic qualities of interrelation and interconnection between the self and the source of all being.

The word *prayer* comes from the Latin *precari,* "to ask earnestly, beg, entreat." This origin suggests two of the most common forms of prayer: petition, asking something for oneself; and intercession, asking something for others. Prayer is a genuinely nonlocal event, not confined to a specific place in space or to a specific moment in time. Prayer reaches outside the here and now; it operates at a distance and outside the present moment. Because prayer is initiated by a mental action, some aspects of our psyche also are genuinely nonlocal. Nonlocality implies infinitude in space and time, because a limited nonlocality is a contradiction in terms. In the West, this infinite aspect of the human psyche has often been referred to as the soul. Empirical evidence for the power of prayer therefore may be seen as indirect evidence for the existence of the soul.

For scientific attempts to assess the effects of prayer and spiritual practices on health, we begin again in the nineteenth century with Sir Francis Galton (1822–1911), an English polymath and nephew of Charles Darwin. Galton's 1872 treatise *Statistical Inquiries into the Efficacy of Prayer* assessed the longevity of people frequently prayed for, such as clergymen, monarchs, and heads of state. He concluded that there was no demonstrable effect of prayer on longevity, but of course his study did not meet current scientific standards. He was successful, however, in promoting the idea that prayer is subject to empirical scientific scrutiny. Galton acknowledged that praying could make a person feel better. In the end he maintained that although his attempts to prove the efficacy of prayer had failed, he could see no good reason to abandon prayer (a bit like Pascal's wager).

THE PROVEN EFFECTIVENESS
OF PRAYER FOR HEALING

Research during the last three decades has made an indelible mark on the way health care professionals think about the role of spirituality in physical, mental, and social health. Hundreds of studies have explored the relations between body and spirit. Most studies have been cross-sectional (the analysis of data collected from a population, or a representative subset, at one specific point in time), but some have also been longitudinal (repeated observations of the same variables over long periods of time, often many decades, in the same sample of people). Many studies document an association between spirituality and lower anxiety, fewer psychotic symptoms, less substance abuse, and better coping mechanisms. Other studies have shown that spirituality and religiosity are clearly associated with longer survival, healthier behaviors, and less distress and are believed to have a positive effect on coping, anxiety, aging, end of life, and cortisol measures of stress.

A 2000 comprehensive review found that two-thirds of nearly 750 studies showed a significant relationship between spiritual involvement and better mental health and greater social support.[7] The review also found that almost all of those who are religious have significantly greater well-being, hope, and optimism compared to those who are not religious. (Note that in this study, the identification of religious people was relating to organized religion, believing in God, and following the rules of a religion, which does not necessarily encompass spirituality in the larger sense that we are using to discuss spiritual healing and spirit.) At Duke University, studies have been conducted examining the effects of religiousness on the course of depression in nearly a thousand hospitalized patients over the age of sixty. Those who used coping mechanisms based on religious practices showed lower levels of depressive symptoms measured at baseline and again at six months after discharge.[8]

Those who practice healing with prayer claim uniformly that the effects are not diminished with distance; therefore, it falls within the nonlocal perspective. Claims about the effectiveness of prayer do not rely on anecdotes or single case studies; numerous controlled studies have validated the nonlocal nature of prayer. Much of this evidence suggests that people who pray, or people involved in compassionate imagery or mental intent, whether or not it is called "prayer," can purposefully affect the physiology of someone else at a distance without the receiver's knowing.

The medical community has recently begun to acknowledge the importance of the association between spirituality and health. Many medical schools now offer courses in religion, spirituality, and health. According to a 1994 survey, 98 percent of hospitalized patients ascribe to a belief in God or some higher power, and 96 percent acknowledge a personal use of prayer to aid in the healing process. In addition, 77 percent of over two hundred hospitalized general medical patients believed that their physicians should consider their spiritual needs. In contrast, only one-third of the patients' family physicians actually discussed spirituality with their patients.[9] Anecdotal accounts of the power of prayer to heal are legion and legendary, and countless books on these subjects are available.

A famous prayer study was published in 1988 by Randolph Byrd, a staff cardiologist at the University of California San Francisco School of Medicine, involving nearly four hundred patients in the coronary care unit who were receiving intercessory prayer. Intercessory prayer was offered by people outside the hospital who were instructed not how to pray, but to pray as they saw fit. In this study, the prayed-for patients did better on several counts: there were fewer deaths in the prayer group; they were less likely to require intubation and ventilator support; they required fewer potent drugs; they experienced a lower incidence of pulmonary edema; and they required cardiopulmonary resuscitation less often.[10]

In 1999, a follow-up study by a different group of researchers attempted to replicate Byrd's findings under stricter experimental conditions, noting that the original research was not completely blinded and was limited to only "prayer-receptive" individuals (fifty-seven of the 450 patients, or only about 12 percent, invited to participate in the study refused to give consent "for personal reasons or religious convictions"). Researchers concluded that "supplementary, remote, blinded, intercessory prayer produced a measurable improvement in the medical outcomes of critically ill patients," and they suggested that "prayer be an effective adjunct to standard medical care."[11]

Other studies have been conducted with intercessory prayer as the intervention for alcohol abuse and dependence, kidney dialysis, and self-esteem. A 2000 longitudinal study of forty patients with painful class II or III rheumatoid arthritis compared the effects of direct-contact intercessory prayer with distant prayer. Persons receiving direct-contact prayer showed significant overall improvement at the one-year follow-up, while the distant prayer group showed no additional benefits.[12]

The benefits of spiritual healing were examined in 120 patients with chronic pain at the Department of Complementary Medicine at the University of Exeter, United Kingdom. Patients were provided either with face-to-face healing thirty minutes per week for eight weeks, with distant healing, or with no healing for the same period of time.

Although subjects in both healing groups, the face-to-face and the distant, reported significantly more "unusual experiences" during the sessions, the clinical results were unclear. It was concluded that a specific effect of face-to-face or distant healing on chronic pain could not be demonstrated over just eight treatment sessions.[13]

Although research problems are difficult to overcome in scientifically evaluating the power of prayer, Byrd's initial prayer study broke significant ground in medical research. Many questions still remain unanswered, and further study is warranted to define the role of intercessory prayer on outcomes and to identify endpoints that best measure efficacy. Nevertheless, validated evidence continues to build concerning the efficacy of prayer.

My friend, physician Larry Dossey, author of the 1993 book *Healing Words: The Power of Prayer and the Practice of Medicine,* maintains that some serious questions arise in the wake of these experiments. The evidence clearly shows that mental activity can be used to influence people nonlocally, at a distance, without their knowledge. Scores of experiments on prayer also show that it can be used to great effect without the subject's awareness. Therefore, the question is whether it is ethical to use these techniques if recipients are unaware that they are being used. This question becomes even more compelling as we consider the possibility that prayer, or any other form of nonlocal mind-to-mind communication, could also potentially be used at a distance to harm people without their knowledge. Institutional review committees that oversee the design of experiments involving humans to ensure their safety have rarely had to consider these types of ethical considerations.

Combining Mind-Body-Spirit Approaches

While evidence continues to mount regarding the efficacy of mind-body approaches used individually, as we have seen in previous chapters, more and more researchers and clinicians are beginning to combine these approaches with spirituality in order to create a synergistic healing process.

Funded by the U.S. Department of Defense, the California Pacific Medical Center conducted a study that examined the outcomes for

181 women with breast cancer. Author Micozzi met with the investigators to discuss how to conduct this study after they had been awarded the research funds to pursue it. Women were randomized to a twelve-week "mind, body, and spirit" support group or to a standard support group. The mind, body, and spirit women were taught meditation, affirmations, visual imagery, and ritual. The standard group combined cognitive-behavioral approaches with group sharing and support. Both interventions were found to be associated with improved quality of life, decreased depression and anxiety, and spiritual well-being, but only the mind-body-spirit group showed significant increases in measures of spiritual integration. At the end of the intervention, the mind-body-spirit group also showed higher satisfaction and had fewer dropouts than the standard group.[14]

A 2003 study consisted of a similar intervention for breast cancer survivors using a mind, body, and spirit self-empowerment program. Over fifty women attended a twelve-week psychospiritual supportive program that included multiple strategies for creating a balance among spiritual, mental, emotional, and physical health. Components included meditation, visualization, guided imagery, affirmations, and dream work. Results showed statistically significant improvements in depression, perceived wellness, quality of life, and spiritual well-being.[15]

BOUNDARY TYPES:
WHO BENEFITS AND WHY

A thin boundary person, almost by definition, finds less of a separation between what is inside and what is "out there." They are generally more susceptible and accepting of spiritual experiences, feelings, and emotions that transcend physical dimensions and physical limits. When boundaries are thin, these experiences come naturally, almost automatically, and sometimes unbidden. For the thick boundary person, genuine belief and practice in religious traditions and the experience of spirituality present a form and place to open to experience outside the body, to which a thick boundary typically closes the door, so to speak. In the right time, place, and circumstances—either in communal observations or in solitary practices of contemplation, mindfulness, and meditation—there is permission for the thick person to open the door to other experiences, feelings, and emotions. With practice and observation the hinge of the door is well oiled and the access comes easily and naturally.

So, we don't attempt to associate the practice and benefits of spirituality to one boundary type or another (and remember, everyone exists somewhere on a spectrum anyway), nor would that be appropriate to do. Spirituality is accessible to everyone; it is typically a question of what path you take.

PART TWO

❦

Hands-On Healing

The first part of this book has addressed mind-body-spirit techniques that work to facilitate healing. Part 2 addresses bodywork and physical manipulations of the body that help the physical body while also having profound effects for healing on mental and spiritual levels.

8

Massage and Bodywork

Ancient civilizations developed forms of manual manipulation of the body, massage, and therapeutic touch similar to techniques used today, including traction (pulling and stretching), rubbing the muscles, and passively moving joints. Today a bodyworker is likely to use his or her hands, and possibly elbows, forearms, and even feet, to directly apply techniques (sometimes called "manual manipulation") to your body for enhancing health and well-being.

There are many different approaches that arise from a broad range of viewpoints. A variety of "lenses" can be used to view the body through structure, function, movement, neural communication, or energetic means. The practitioner's perspective and skills influence which application he or she chooses for you and determine which techniques to employ to best achieve your goals. Speed of movement of the hand on the skin, the depth of pressure used, whether lubrication is employed, or whether the hand even contacts the body combine to shape the desired outcomes for a given session.

The origin of the earliest forms of manipulative therapy is not known. It was recorded that Hippocrates was skilled in the use of manipulation and taught it in his school of medicine more than two thousand years ago. Ancient Chinese drawings tell of the use of manual therapies, and there are even prehistoric depictions of manual therapies by early humans ("cavemen") prior to written historical records. Massage therapy is also documented in the writings of ancient Chinese medicine. In China, the history of the manual therapy known as *tui na* (or *tuina*) predates the development of the metallurgical technology necessary to produce the needles used for acupuncture. *Tui* means "to push," and *na* means "to lift and squeeze." The term is found in Chinese medical classics dating back to 2000 BCE. *Amna* is a practice of traditional Japanese massage from which modern shiatsu is said to have derived. It is thought to be of Chinese origin, developing from tui na. *Romi-romi* is the term used by Polynesians to describe methods of manual healing that use certain massage techniques and manipulations. Hawaiians refer to the same technique as *lomi-lomi*. Translations have to do with rubbing, pressing, lifting, pounding, and stretching.

European styles are said to have originated with the work of Per Henrik Ling (1766–1839) of Sweden and Johan Georg Mezger (1839–1909) of Holland. The movement system developed by Ling, which included massage, was coined the Swedish Gymnastic Movements and he developed the curriculum of the Royal Central Gymnastic Institute founded in 1813. Ling has been known in the Western world to have created "Swedish massage"; however, this is an error. Ling was Swedish, and his movement system included certain massage techniques, but they were not the techniques we have come to know as Swedish or classic massage. Ling *attempted* to develop massage as an actual medical therapy in the West. He arranged physical exercises and the elements of traditional massage technique according to the principles of anatomy and physiology, as they were then understood. Ling's system became known as remedial gymnastics. Ling popularized massage and particularly the idea of using passive movements, where the therapist manipulates your body while you are in a state of relaxation, without intentional or voluntary movement.

Dutch practitioner Mezger is credited with providing the French names to denote the basic strokes of Swedish massage. Born the year of Ling's death, Mezger and his followers organized massage into a recognizable form using different procedures. They gave these techniques French names, like *pétrissage* (kneading), *tapotement* (slapping), and *effleurage* (stroking). Massage combined with heat and exercise became a basic technique used by physical therapists during the polio epidemics of the nineteenth and early twentieth centuries. During the early twentieth century, various books on the benefits of massage were published, including the 1929 classic *The Art of Massage,* still in publication, by John Harvey Kellogg (also known for packaging "healthy" breakfast cereals and for advocating the "nature cure").

Physiotherapy and physical therapy made many advances in the treatment of neurological diseases during the twentieth century. The requirement for more higher education by practitioners followed, as is usual whenever experts begin to specialize in a particular practice. It became required for physical therapists to learn neuroanatomy, neurophysiology, and kinesiology. Despite the addition of more scientific perspectives, massage practice declined, as the new requirements and restrictions meant there were fewer practitioners available to conduct basic daily practice. During the 1950s, modern devices and techniques using machines came into vogue, such as galvanic stimulation, automated traction, and other treatments performed by technology, not the healing hands of people. These large-scale "improvements" led to further declines in the personalized and labor-intensive use of massage in physical therapy. The machines could be effective and saved time, by certain measures, but a vital personal element of health and healing was lost to the technology that also generally overtook and totally transformed medicine during the twentieth century. One of the most ancient healing arts, using personal touch, was being lost.

In the years that followed, the practice of massage became confined to health clubs and spas, as well as escort services (this was not a "happy ending" for the use of massage as a healing art). Massage practitioners were referred to as "masseuses" and "masseurs." Training was offered only in a small number of schools. Massage training ultimately fell under the domain of vocational education, along with ophthalmic dispensers and bartenders.

During the physical fitness craze of the 1970s, massage again began to gain interest and use as an effective natural health approach. Today, there are hundreds of schools, some offering associate of occupational studies (AOS) degree programs. Other educational institutions throughout America are developing similar programs in higher education (see "Finding a Practitioner" on page 144).

The 1950 American Medical Association's *Handbook of Physical Medicine and Rehabilitation* says of massage, "There is probably no other measure of equal known value in the entire armamentarium of medicine which is so inadequately understood and utilized by the profession as a whole."[1] Currently, massage therapy, despite its obvious health benefits, still remains somewhat outside the core of standard medical practice in terms of routine doctor referrals, insurance coverage, reimbursement, and medical treatment protocols. However, Medicare does cover massage two times a week for various medical conditions for people over sixty-five, due to its proven effectiveness. When I (Micozzi) ran the Thomas Jefferson Center for Integrative Medicine ten years ago, we offered many different natural therapies that were generally not covered or reimbursed by health insurance. To help provide cash flow to the clinic, we were able to build a massage program around the twice-weekly Medicare payments for senior patients. Since we were located right inside a tertiary-care hospital (in the "belly of the beast"), there were plenty of older patients who needed and benefited from this simple, safe, effective, low-cost therapy. So that was one therapy we actually managed to *integrate* into an integrative health care setting.

WHAT IS MASSAGE?

The Latin word *massa* means "to knead." Today, the English word *massage* describes a way of touching that moves the skin and muscle layers around and against the bones using a kneading action. Massage therapy, or therapeutic massage, is the practice of using skilled movement and touch for the purposes of reducing your pain associated with disease, injury, or stress. The scope of massage practice may include muscular rehabilitation and disease prevention.

A massage may consist of any or all of eight components. They are all major aspects of relating to and engaging with the body. Many of these you will recognize from the chapters on relaxation, stress reduction, and other mind-body therapies in the previous section of the book.

Breathing (tracking, directing, pacing) engages your mechanism of respiration, which creates energetic waves that impact every system of your body.

Cognitive (visualizing, inquiring, intending, focusing transmitting) consists of tools for assessment, enhancement, modification, and change.

Energy (sensing, intuiting, balancing) is effective in detecting distortions and assisting your body to establish balance.

Compression (pressing/pushing, squeezing/pinching, twisting/wringing) applies a force to your body, reducing the space within and between structures and pressing fluid out.

Expansion (pulling, lifting, rolling) opens up space within and between your body's structures, bringing fluid into them.

Kinetics (holding/supporting, mobilizing, letting go/dropping, stabilizing) focuses on the movement relationships among segments of your body.

Oscillation (vibrating, shaking, striking) initiates waves by applying intermittent or continuous vibratory contact.

Gliding (sliding/planing, rubbing) follows the contours of your skin, muscle, tendon, ligament, bone, and fascial layers.

For you as an individual, the practitioner blends these basic elements to achieve the desired changes within your myofascial tissues. You can experience massage as a few basic movement techniques or including all eight components, as above. Either way, the practitioner moves seamlessly from one technique to another. The therapist's deliberate and intuitive decisions are made in the moment by what is discovered and felt within your tissues and body.

Muscle-Energy Techniques

Muscle-energy techniques fall into the category of neuromuscular therapy. These techniques require your active participation through a series of controlled muscle contractions. The techniques include active, isolated stretching.

Muscle-energy technique (MET) can be applied directly or indirectly to your individual muscles or to your muscle groups.[2] MET may be applied directly toward the barrier to normal motion of the muscle or in an attempt to lengthen a shortened or spastic muscle. This technique is based on the principle of reciprocal inhibition, which states that a muscle (e.g., a flexor) reflexively relaxes as its opposite muscle, or antagonist (the associated extensor), contracts. Conversely, if your muscle is in spasm and is contracted against resistance and then relaxed, the effect often results in increased range of motion, or reduction of the motion barrier.[3]

This technique is one of the few "active" techniques in manual therapy; that is to say, you, the patient, do most of the work. A distinction of MET is the amount of effort exerted by the patient. Usually, less than 20 percent of the total strength of the muscle is brought to bear during the interval of contraction. Another way of demonstrating this idea is through the "one-finger rule": the amount of force necessary is the force needed to move a single finger of the practitioner when the practitioner lightly resists the contraction. This is distinguished from the technique often used in physical therapy, which employs a maximal muscle contraction and may expose you to the risk of injury. A therapist's thorough knowledge of muscle attachments and their motion vectors is necessary to apply MET safely and effectively.

Neuromuscular Techniques

Neuromuscular therapy (NMT) involves more precise treatment of the soft tissues of a joint or region that is experiencing pain. It is a medically oriented technique, primarily used for the treatment of chronic pain or as a treatment for recent (but not acute) trauma or injury. It can also be applied to prevent injury or to enhance performance.

NMT emerged on two continents almost at the same time, but the two forms had little connection to each other until recently. In the early twentieth century, European "neuromuscular technique" emerged, and for the last several decades it has been developing through the teachings of Leon Chaitow, DO. The practice of North American "neuromuscular therapy," as it is known here, derives from a variety of sources, including chiropractic, myofascial trigger-point therapy (as developed by Janet Travell), and massage therapy (as developed by Judith DeLany). Over the last decade, Chaitow and DeLany combined the two methods and integrated the European and American versions.[4] NMT continues to evolve, with many people teaching the techniques worldwide.

One of the main features of NMT is a step-by-step protocol that addresses all muscles of a region. Like osteopathy, neuromuscular therapy uses the idea of somatic dysfunction when describing what is found during examination of your body. Body dysfunction is usually characterized by having tender tissues and limited and/or painful range of motion, caused by connective tissue changes, ischemia (lack of blood flow), nerve compression, and posture disturbances. Any of these conditions can result from trauma, stress, and repetitive microtrauma from stress due to repetitive work and recreation-related patterns of activity. Identification and treatment of trigger points is key to this therapy. Trigger points are highly irritable nodules within your myofascial tissues that radiate pain to a defined target zone when provoked by applied pressure or needling. Consideration is also given to nutrition, hydration, hormonal balance, breathing patterns, and numerous other factors that impact your health.

The European and American versions both examine for taut bands often associated with trigger points and use applied pressure to treat the pain-producing nodules. American NMT offers a more systematic method of examination and treatment. European methods use less detail in palpation of deeper structures and incorporate positional release and other methods for the deeper treatment. European methods also focus significantly more on superficial tissue texture changes. Both European and American NMT use hydrotherapy (water), temperature (hot and cold applications), movement, and self-applied (home-care) therapies. Both suggest homework to encourage your participation in the recovery process, which might include doing stretching, changes in habits of use, and alterations in lifestyle that help you eliminate perpetuating factors. You may also be offered education to increase awareness of your posture and movements in work and recreational settings and healthy nutritional choices.

What You Experience

Your superficial tissues are treated before deeper layers, and proximal (closer) areas of an extremity are treated before distal (farther) regions. Every muscle in the region is assessed, not just those whose patterns are consistent with your pain or that are thought to be the cause of the problem. This approach also helps reveal muscles you may be using to compensate for those that are painful, dysfunctional, or weak.

The first aim is to increase blood flow and soften connecting tissue. Although gliding strokes are often the first choice, sometimes tissue manipulation (sliding the tissues between the thumb and finger to create shearing) works better. Hot packs might be used to further encourage softening of your muscles and connective tissues. Then gliding strokes and manipulation may be repeated, alternating with the application of heat.

Once your tissues have become softer and more pliable, the practitioner palpates for taut bands. Taut bands have select fibers locked into a shortened position and vary in diameter from being as small as a toothpick to larger than a finger. At the center of the band there is often a thicker, denser area that is associated with central trigger-point pain formation.

Once the fiber center is located, the region is evaluated for a trigger point. Pressure is applied until a degree of resistance (like an "elastic barrier") is felt. Sufficient pressure is applied to match the tension that provokes or intensifies your pain referred to the target zone. The applied pressure is monitored, so that what you feel as the person being massaged is no more than a moderate level of discomfort (7 on a scale of 1 to 10). Although you may feel some tenderness in the area that is being pressed, usually focus is directed onto the pain, tingling, numbness, burning, or other sensation in the associated target zone of your trigger point. These well-documented, common target zones are usually distant from the location of the trigger point itself and the zones of referral are predictable.

Orthopedic Massage

Orthopedic massage (OM) is a comprehensive assessment and treatment system that may incorporate several techniques. It has broad applications based on your symptoms and can be incorporated into relaxation massage, sports injury care, and a diverse range of medical settings, as well as advanced rehabilitative therapy. Using these modalities requires skills in orthopedic assessment, variability of treatment, and advanced knowledge of pain, injuries, and, in some cases, clinical protocols for rehabilitation.[5]

OM drew its roots from sports massage, which emerged in the United States in the 1970s and 1980s. Practice settings are as diverse as the application itself and include private practices, physical therapy clinics, medical settings, chiropractic offices, spas, and sport facilities.

Whitney Lowe, author of the orthopedic massage protocols, describes the value of orthopedic massage as follows, "Assessment is at the very foundation of orthopedic massage. It is paramount to identify the tissues most likely at the root of a problem for effective management of soft tissue pain and injuries. . . . Skilled orthopedic massage therapists have good knowledge of what tissues are involved and which therapeutic techniques would best treat those tissues. Thus, they are not limited by their 'technique toolbag' and can employ established, as well as newly developed, techniques and methods, and hence are adaptable to the patient's condition. Their advanced education and knowledge leads to outcome-based therapeutic treatments and effective solutions."[6]

OM and NMT have long been established as successful interventions that can deliver highly effective results. They should not be confused with what is known as "medical massage," a term that has become popular in the last fifteen years as a result of the aim of national massage organizations to standardize protocols being integrated into medical communities. There is no one style of massage that comprises medical massage. OM and NMT practitioners perform outcome-based massage targeted to your specific condition(s), in this sense fitting within a broad definition of "medical massage." However, "orthopedic massage" and "neuromuscular therapy" better define the specific degree of training such therapists have received and the protocols they use.

Myofascial Release

Myofascial release is based on the principle of piezoelectricity: a low load (gentle pressure) applied slowly will allow a viscoelastic medium (fascia) to elongate. Also known as "myofascial therapy" or "myofascial trigger point therapy," myofascial release is a technique used to eliminate pain and restore motion. To stimulate the stretch reflex in muscles, it applies gentle, sustained pressure into the myofascial connective tissue restrictions that cause muscle immobility and pain caused by trauma, inflammatory responses, or surgical procedures.

Fascia is a thin, tough, elastic type of connective tissue that wraps around most structures within the human body, including muscle, supporting and protecting your body's structures. Osteopathic theory proposes that this soft tissue can become restricted due to disease, overuse, trauma, infectious agents, or inactivity, often resulting in pain, muscle tension, and diminished blood flow. A myofascial release treatment is performed directly on your skin without oils, creams, or machinery. This enables the therapist to accurately detect fascial restrictions and apply the appropriate amount of sustained pressure to facilitate release of the fascia. Myofascial techniques can be passive (you stay completely relaxed) or active (you provide resistance as asked), with direct and indirect techniques used in each session.

Hydrotherapy and Cryotherapy

Hydrotherapy is a term used to describe the therapeutic use of water in the form of hot or cold applications or immersions, while cryotherapy (cold therapy) refers to the use of ice or ice massage.

Different temperatures, hot or cold, influence muscles and nerve activities. Massage therapy and bodywork may incorporate hot towels or compresses as well as cold packs at the discretion of the therapist. You can also learn to use hot or cold at home to help your pain. Make sure the hot application is not too hot (try touching and brushing it against the wrist to make sure the temperature is not uncomfortable). For cold, do not go below the temperature of ice and do not leave in place for more than a few minutes. If any temperature, hot or cold, feels uncomfortable, discontinue immediately.

Chinese Tui Na

Chinese tu nai is used to influence qi through physical massage and manipulation. Qi, the body's vital energy, is a universal force that permeates all living matter. It is manifest in five separate elements or phases: fire, wood, metal, water, and earth. The organs of the body correspond to each phase and are categorized accordingly. Qi flows through all the meridians, or channels, and each meridian and its associated organ has daily strong and weak periods. When the flow of qi is impeded in any channel, that organ or function may become dysfunctional, or imbalanced, resulting in disorders and symptoms such as pain.

Tui na combine soft tissue, visceral, and joint manipulations. Typically, you lie on a table or are seated. Soft-tissue techniques are applied to your limbs, trunk, and head, preceding joint mobilization, to prepare your joints for movement and to relax the surrounding musculature. The techniques stimulate local blood flow, venous and lymphatic drainage, and the flow of qi. These soft-tissue techniques include the following:

- pressing, using the thumbs, elbows, or palms
- squeezing, using the whole hand or finger-thumb combination
- kneading, a circular pressing technique, using the thumbs, heel of the hand, elbow, or forearm
- rubbing, a high-frequency technique, using the palms, heels of the hands (chafing), or forearms
- stroking (like the Swedish massage technique *effleurage*), moving the hand over the skin in a long stroke, in one direction only
- thumb rocking, for deep penetration of acupuncture points
- plucking, a transverse friction-type technique
- rolling, using the back of the hand to roll over the skin and underlying tissue
- percussion (like the Swedish massage technique *tapotement*), which includes pummeling with the fists, striking with the heels of the hands, and pounding with cupped hands

Joint manipulative techniques include the following:

- shaking, in which traction is applied to your limb, and it is shaken ten to twenty times with high-velocity, low-amplitude movements

- flexion and extension, primarily applied to the hinge joints, such as elbows and knees, using both high- and low-velocity techniques designed to engage a motion barrier but not to challenge it (in addition, in some of these techniques a thumb is simultaneously applied to an acupuncture point to open a meridian)
- rotation, an articulatory technique used for the ankles, wrists, hips, and shoulders (practitioners of tui na do not apply this technique to the neck)
- pushing and pulling, a low-velocity technique designed to directly engage a motion barrier, with a counterforce applied by the opposing hand in the opposite direction
- stretching, a general low-velocity flexion-extension technique used to loosen the joints of the spine
- thrust, used on the spinal joints in a manner similar to that of osteopathic and chiropractic methods

Tui na can be applied to virtually anyone. The contraindications include skin lesions or infection, skin or lymphatic cancer, and osteoporosis. It is recommended that the low back and abdomen be avoided if the person is pregnant.

Zen Shiatsu

Developed by Shizuto Masunaga, Zen shiatsu is one of several forms of Asian bodywork that arose as a synthesis of acupuncture and anma, traditional Japanese massage. Shiatsu (Japanese for "finger pressure") is a Japanese bodywork modality that approaches the human form in both health and disease according to ancient Asian beliefs and methodologies. Shiatsu directly affects the energy meridian systems that govern the organs of the body, as is delineated in Chinese medicine and applied in acupuncture (see chapter 10). The manipulation of *qi* (or *chi*), the life force, by skillful and intuitive contact of the *tsubos* (points) along the meridians forms the basis of treatment. Your individual needs are assessed by evaluation before, during, and after the session.

During the eighteenth and nineteenth centuries, anma became more associated with carnal pleasure, and as a result it lost its place as a therapeutic practice. However, a number of recent studies have re-examined the therapeutic benefits of anma.[7] Shiatsu further diverged and became systematized in the twentieth century, with the Nippon Shiatsu School opening in the late 1940s. Today, shiatsu is practiced worldwide in a number of settings with strong roots in energy-based medicine. The physical nature of its practice offers a quality more like massage than typical energy work. Shiatsu can be applied for a more energetic approach when you cannot tolerate much movement against your body.

THE PROVEN EFFECTIVENESS OF BODYWORK AND MASSAGE

The benefits of massage are both physiological and psychological, and results depend on which technique is used and the corresponding effects on your tissues, organs, or entire body system. In general, massage and bodywork

- improve the circulation of blood and lymph
- reduce lymphatic obstruction
- speed recovery of fatigued muscles
- improve joint range of motion
- induce muscle relaxation
- break down joint adhesions
- improve neuromuscular function after spinal-cord injury
- improve breathing and ventilation
- result in transient increase in sympathetic nervous tone
- change skin temperature
- transiently raise endorphins
- assist in growth and development
- improve responses to stress in the brain

Skin is the primary organ through which all nurturing originally occurs. When receiving massage you may enter a hypnagogic state of deep relaxation resembling sleep. This effect may reduce psychological defenses, allowing you to feel cared for and nurtured. Accordingly, massage reduces anxiety.

Anxiety and Panic Attacks

General massage is great for relaxing your muscles and decreasing all forms of anxiety. An extreme form of anxiety, a panic attack is a sudden period of intense fear or apprehension, accompanied by bodily or cognitive symptoms. A true panic attack may last anywhere from minutes to hours and can include increased perspiration, a feeling of terror, difficulty breathing or shortness of breath, uncontrollable yelling or screaming, tightness in the chest, dizziness, uncontrollable muscle trembling or contraction, fear of dying, fear of losing control, thoughts of going insane, out-of-body experiences, and other similar sensations related to the flight-or-fight response of the autonomic nervous system. The panic reaction to stress can begin at an early age and may disappear in adulthood, only to return during periods of great stress, or it may arise only in adulthood. Most people can recover from a panic attack without medication; however, if panic attacks occur frequently and appear to worsen over time, additional attention should be sought.

Persons pursuing massage therapy for panic attacks can benefit from the general nurturing and soothing effects massage has on the mind and nervous system. The treatment should consist of gentle strokes performed in rhythmic, predictable patterns. Deep and continuous breathing should be encouraged and monitored throughout the session.

Back Pain

Back pain may occur in the musculoskeletal tissues of the spine, such as ligaments, facets, and intrinsic muscles. All of these structures, including the intervertebral disks, can be pain-sensitive. Pain arising from these areas appears to be caused not by neurological problems or nerve root compression, but rather by inflammatory or degenerative processes resulting from injury, disease, or normal wear and tear. An orthopedic assessment assists the practitioner in formulating a unique treatment plan for the person and becomes the basis for noting progress. For pain that is not due to cancer, massage lowers pain intensity scores and reduces consumption of pain drugs.[8]

Myofascial pain syndrome refers to pain induced when your muscles and soft tissues are inflamed and pressure is applied. Pressure applied directly on an active trigger point in the shoulder-blade muscle, for example, often elicits pain in the midback and along the spine. Posture and mechanical problems contribute to the formation of trigger points as nodules of fibrous tissue that have become ischemic (having lessened blood flow). Trigger points also are related to muscular spasm "holding patterns" and the creation of a pain/spasm/pain cycle. Treatment of trigger points uses a combination of direct digital pressure followed by thorough passive stretching.

Post-traumatic pain can be the result of physical injury, whether resulting from an accident, an assault, poisoning, near-drowning, or recovery from surgery. Psychological trauma also must be addressed because some degree of mental anguish coincides with post-traumatic pain. For treatment to be fully successful, you should pursue help on all levels by participating in physical therapy that includes massage as well as psychological, emotional, or spiritual counseling.

Carpal Tunnel Syndrome

Carpal tunnel syndrome is a compression of the median nerve of the arm where it passes through the carpal tunnel at the wrist and through the surface of the hand. Causes can include the narrowing of the space between the carpal wrist bones and the transverse carpal ligament, and/or looseness of the carpal ligaments as a result of repetitive motion, strain, and maintaining a static wrist position. Impingement of the median nerve causes a sharp shooting pain that starts at the proximal wrist flexors and extends into the wrist. The pain often begins after activity and can persist to disturb sleep. Chronic impingement can cause atrophy of the thumb muscle. Some of the commonly associated areas of neurovascular compression, such as the cervical, interscalene, subclavicular, pectoral, cubital, and ulnar nerves, should also be explored as contributing factors.

In addition, treatment of carpal tunnel pain must address the muscle spasm holding patterns that can develop. The shrug mechanism, in which the shoulders are tightened and uplifted, is the most common type of muscular contraction and can limit recovery if not treated. The other holding pattern is the tendency to "splint the arm" by tensing the muscles of the upper chest, shoulder, and/or arm, resulting in muscular spasms, which impede circulation in the armpit and interfere with the healing process. Treatment should include general massage and lymphatic drainage techniques to prepare for deeper pressure. Myofascial release and specific nerve release techniques are used in areas where nerves are compromised or compressed. Squeezing the ulna and radius at the wrist during passive movement improves ligament tone and helps restore the carpal arch. Passive mobilization of the neck, shoulder, elbow, and wrist ensures complete coverage of related areas.

A related condition is ulnar neuropathy, where the ulnar nerve becomes trapped or pinched due to some physiological abnormalities. This condition responds to the kinds of treatment outlined for carpal tunnel syndrome, with the addition of ulnar nerve release. This technique involves thrusting with a "plucking" motion the flexor carpi ulnaris muscle from the medial surface of the ulna, from just below the elbow through the ulnar tunnel and the hypothenar muscle of the thumb.

Radial tunnel syndrome (posterior interosseous nerve syndrome) is caused by increased pressure on the radial nerve as it travels from the upper arm (the brachial plexus) to the hand and wrist. Techniques that thrust the extensor carpi radialis longus (one of the five main muscles that control movements at the wrist, which starts on the lateral side of the humerus and attaches to the base of the metacarpal of the index finger) and the extensor carpi radialis brevis muscle (the muscle in the forearm that acts to extend and abduct the wrist) medially from the posterior surface of the radius should be performed from the proximal (close to the point of attachment) to the distal (away from the point of attachment) portions of the bone. Vigorous rubbing along the interosseus membrane (the fibrous sheet that connects the radius and the ulna) is also helpful.

Thoracic outlet syndrome involves an interference of proper

pulsation and blood flow through the subclavian artery as it passes through the interscalene triangle of the upper body, shoulder, and neck. This condition can result from a variety of mechanical impingements and bony compressions. Myofascial release of neurovascular compression at the interscalene triangle, the subclavicular area, and the pectoralis minor muscle has been quite successful in treatment.

Headache

A comfortable, quiet, dimly lit environment is helpful during a massage treatment to relieve a headache. When a migraine is already in progress, even the most gentle massage may be too disturbing. However, most headaches, including migraines, are relieved or greatly reduced by massaging the skull, neck, and facial structures (such as sinuses). Shiatsu point pressure on the cranium can quell even the worst pounding headache in minutes. The relief from pain may last for hours or days, depending on the cause. Massage provides pain relief and also improves mood.

A relaxation response is achieved by gently stroking the head and neck in rhythmic patterns. When suffering from a headache, you can participate in the relaxation response by breathing slowly and deeply during the session. Guided imagery can be helpful if you who find it difficult to release muscle tension (see chapter 4). Lymphatic drainage, traction of the cervical vertebrae, and rubbing the sides and back of the head reduce muscle tension and fluid retention. Gentle percussions promote drainage of the sinuses to reduce sinus pain. Massage of the abdomen, the lower extremities, and reflex points on the feet also has been effective as part of a more complete approach to the treatment of headache.

There have been several studies on massage for pain relief, representing more than five hundred patients. As judged by reduced pain, reduced need for analgesics, and improved physical functioning, these studies suggest massage may be beneficial for chronic pain conditions including tension headache, migraine with aura, postconcussive headache, nonspecific low-back pain, nonspecific neck pain, inflammatory joint pain, and regional muscle pain.[9]

Insomnia

Sleep disorders, including difficulty sleeping and insufficient sleep, are often associated with chronic pain, anxiety, and dietary factors. Ideally, for this condition, massage treatment should be given late in the day or even just before bedtime (depending on how well you know that massage practitioner). Gentle, predictable, repetitive strokes can induce sleep. Massage of the face, spine, and feet has a particularly hypnotic effect on the central nervous system.

Irritable Bowel Syndrome

A true mind-body disorder that is amenable to massage therapy and bodywork, IBS is becoming more common, affecting up to 15 percent of the U.S. population.[10] The more people know about it and talk about it, the more comfortable sufferers are in seeking help.

It's critical you choose the right kind of help. And it's not just people with diagnosed IBS who need to be concerned. Irritable bowel syndrome (IBS) and its related symptoms may be a warning sign for those who don't make necessary dietary and lifestyle changes. In fact, IBS is a prime example of how the mind and body are connected. It's no surprise that the people who experience chronic gastrointestinal pain or discomfort often have a history of childhood trauma such as physical or sexual abuse, parental divorce, major illness or accident, or death of a loved one. It's the body's expression of the mind's suffering. IBS also runs in families, so biomedical scientists are quick to claim some kind of genetic basis, but lifestyle factors run in families just as much as genes do.

A common denominator among people suffering from this ailment is low serotonin levels. Serotonin, a chemical that relates to thoughts and feelings, is a key neurotransmitter found in the brain; however, 95 percent of it is found in the neuroendocrine tissue of the gut!

When IBS progresses to an inflammatory bowel disease like Crohn's, treatment can be a lifelong process. For many sufferers, conventional treatments offer little relief. Experts recommend a variety of CAM approaches as a powerful treatment.

Our colleague, Joyce Frye, DO, who has contributed several chapters to Micozzi's medical textbooks over the years, was associated with the Center for Integrative Medicine at the University of Maryland School of Medicine. She was interviewed on this topic. "It's not a question of if you should use these alternative and complementary therapies," she emphasized. "It's a question of using them correctly." As Dr. Frye related, "The first goal is to treat the underlying imbalance that has caused a problem, so we can allow the body to heal itself. The second goal is to provide symptom relief in the meantime."[11]

One of the best things about CAM therapies is that they are safe and unlikely to interfere with your conventional medical treatment. What's more, they can actually help you replace essential vitamins and minerals your body is losing because of the disease.

Although it has no clear direct effect on Crohn's disease, massage is a popular stress reducer. If you experience the relaxation that comes from massage, ask your doctor for specific guidelines based on your medical condition, including whether the massage therapist should completely avoid your abdomen and how light or deep the massage should be.

Muscle Cramps

A muscle cramp is a type of sustained muscle contraction caused in part by a disturbance in blood and lymph flow. Cramps tend to occur during periods of rest. Dehydration, faulty alignment, microscopic tears, and poor walking or running habits can all contribute to cramping. Scars resulting from previous injuries can also interfere with normal circulation.

During a severe cramp, the therapist can alternate techniques and use gentle tapping to release muscle spasms, which is generally successful for pain relief. Once the cramp subsides, kneading the muscles promotes better circulation. As soon as it can be tolerated, the area should be rubbed, followed by passive stretching of the muscles, nerves, and fascia connective tissues in the affected area. Stretching facilitates the optimal flow of lymph and blood through the tissues. You can also learn to use these techniques yourself when stricken by a cramp.

Neuralgia

Neuralgia—nerve pain—is often a symptom of muscular atrophy or hypertrophy, which may be further aggravated by unhealthy blood chemistry. Viral infection also can produce neuralgic pain. The nerves most commonly affected by neuralgia are the trigeminal (third cranial) nerve of the head and face, the sciatic nerve, and the brachial nerves of the upper arms. Myofascial release and nerve release techniques effectively alleviate pain, but only temporarily in some cases. Myofascial release and percussion along the courses of the affected nerves are extremely helpful.

BOUNDARY TYPES: WHO BENEFITS AND WHY

Boundary types are about how the mind influences the body. We tested and observed them with respect to what we have called the "super seven" therapies (from thin to thick): hypnosis, acupuncture, biofeedback, imagery and visualization, relaxation and stress reduction, and meditation and yoga, all of which we covered in the preceding chapters.

These "mind-body" approaches work with the mind to influence the body (keeping in mind of course that the mind and body are connected—it is just a question of where you start). But there are also therapies that work primarily with the body to influence the mind.

One influence of body type is determining your susceptibility to manifesting stress as one particular medical condition or another. Boundary types, conversely, help determine which therapies work better for your type than others. Bodywork and massage are very powerful physical techniques performed on the body by a professional practitioner for alleviating stress and promoting relaxation—essentially using the body to influence the mind.

Boundaries are about what you hold inside versus what is outside. The massage practitioner is an outside agent working with your body to influence your mind. Massage is a powerful technique that works across the boundary spectrum. But here is where it can be tricky.

A thin boundary person may be very open to the effects of touch on his or her body but may even be too sensitive; touch, at first may bring up uncomfortable physical sensations and emotional states. Massage may be too painful to the touch with a thin boundary person. There is also an idea (and scientific evidence) that memories, especially emotional experiences, are held or stored not just in the mind, but also in the tissues of the body. Thin boundaries may allow such emotions to easily come to the surface during bodywork and massage, which may result in distress.

The therapist adjusts her or his approach among the various techniques described in this chapter to suit the individual, from light touch and soft strokes to deeper tissue massage. It is essential for you to give feedback to the therapist at all times about what is, or is not, sensitive, uncomfortable, or painful. It is like biofeedback except that in this case *you* are the biofeedback device!

Those with thick boundaries may not like the idea of massage because they don't like being touched by a "stranger" and are not comfortable with being disrobed in a stranger's presence. They are more comfortable keeping boundaries between themselves, their bodies, and the outside world. They like to keep what is out there, out there. However, with an open mind, the therapist can work with you to adjust techniques and design sessions that are more appropriate, that are suited to your comfort zone, and that feel beneficial to you.

There is a powerful old saying that the mind is a terrible thing to waste. When it comes to your boundary types, the body (and bodywork and massage) is a terrible thing to waste in order to gain benefits for the mind. The entire body can be like an organ of consciousness. You can learn to play this organ by yourself as the musician, or you can learn to work with a bodywork or massage therapist who can play your body like an instrument.

FINDING A PRACTITIONER

The American Massage Therapy Association estimates that as of 2015 there were between 300,000 and 350,000 massage practitioners in the United States alone who provide massages to over thirty-nine million adults (about 18 percent of the population) and represent a $12.1 billion industry.[12] More Americans are seeking and utilizing massage therapy than ever before, and 91 percent of those who do find that massage can be effective in reducing pain.[13] Hospital-based massage is on the rise as well; in 2011, 40 percent of hospitals offer one or more alternative therapies, including massage therapy, an increase of more than 33 percent since 2007.[14] In a 2006 survey, the hospitals surveyed indicated that they used massage for the following reasons and patient groups:[15]

- stress management and comfort (71 percent)
- staff stress management (67 percent)
- pain management (67 percent)
- cancer patients (52 percent)
- improving mobility and movement (52 percent)
- pregnant women (51 percent)
- part of physical therapy (50 percent)
- hospice and end-of-life care (37 percent)
- edema (33 percent)
- infants (24 percent)
- postoperative care (25 percent)
- preoperative care (17 percent)

The number of American adults who are discussing massage therapy with their doctor or other health care provider outside of the hospital setting is steadily growing as well. A variety of health care providers are recommending massage therapy to their patients and clients. As of July 2015, among patients who discussed massage therapy with their doctors and health care providers, 69 percent of the health care providers either referred them to a massage therapist or encouraged them to get a massage—54 percent of physicians recommended it, as did 37 percent physical therapists and 46 percent of chiropractors.[16]

The number of massage and shiatsu training programs has grown exponentially in recent decades, in part because of an increasing public demand for more natural approaches to health care. A number of regulating bodies govern the practice of massage and bodywork.

Currently, the national educational standard for massage therapy education consists of five hundred hours of training, and there is a trend toward increasing this number. In the past decade, programs providing 1,000 to 1,200 hours of training and associate degree programs (equivalent to two-year college programs) have become more common. Surveys conducted by the Associated Bodywork and Massage Professionals (ABMP) show continuous and rapid increases in the number of new massage training programs, particularly within the college career arena.

Massage therapy and bodywork schools have a fairly standardized curriculum; it includes communication skills, Eastern and Western bodywork modalities and philosophies, anatomy, physiology, pathology, kinesiology, business practices, ethics, and first aid/CPR. In addition to classroom studies, students gain experiential knowledge by participating in supervised clinical internships. Some schools and colleges require internships as well, which generally take place in hospitals, hospices, assisted-care facilities, athletic departments, and corporations. And massage therapy is not just provided in hospitals and in private treatment offices; increasingly it is being provided in the open, in full view at airports, events, fairs, and even shopping malls. It seems the more virtual our world becomes, the more we seek the human touch to maintain a healthy balance.

The number of states that regulate massage therapy increased from fourteen in 1989 to thirty-eight in 2007, and many of the remaining states have introduced legislation to do so. The increase in regulation of the profession began in the 1990s, when the American Massage Therapy Association formed the National Certification Board for Therapeutic Massage and Bodywork to foster high standards of ethical and professional practice. Support for regulation grew as more practitioners viewed licensing as a way to further legitimize a profession that was at one time associated with sexual services. Many states still have ordinances that require massage therapists be tested for AIDS and other sexually transmitted diseases and receive regular physicals. This antiquated system that attempted to curtail and control prostitution is vanishing as the massage therapy profession asserts ownership and protection of the practice of massage therapy.

There are a number of professional massage and bodywork organizations and associations in the United States and Canada. The American Massage Therapy Association (AMTA), founded in 1943, now has more than fifty-six thousand members. The organization's website (www.amtamassage.org) has a "find a massage therapist" locator to help you find a qualified practitioner. The AMTA supports its members by providing continuing education through regional and national conferences and conventions and by offering liability insurance. Some massage and bodywork schools are accredited by organizations like the Accrediting Commission of Career Schools and Colleges of Technology, the Accrediting Council for Continuing Education and Training, the Council on Occupational Education, and the Commission on Massage Therapy Accreditation.

Practitioners with other credentials also may offer massage. Soft-tissue manipulation may be included in chiropractic care. Osteopathic physicians, once uniformly trained in soft-tissue manipulation, may or may not incorporate this therapy into their medical practices. Swedish massage technique is used in the standard "back rub" taught in nursing schools. Physical therapists employ Swedish massage, trigger-point stimulation, and myofascial manipulation. Podiatrists may provide foot massage. Cosmetologists give facial, scalp, and neck massages. Many other bodywork techniques may properly fall under the category of soft-tissue manipulation, such as reflexology, Feldenkrais, Rolfing, and acupressure, and may be practiced without regulation, although practitioners of these modalities receive training and may be credentialed within their respective fields.

9

Chiropractic

Chiropractic—spinal manual therapy—is a technique for adjusting the alignment of the spinal vertebrae and other joints that offers you a safe and effective way to alleviate many types of musculoskeletal pain. It is provided by all chiropractic doctors, many physical therapists, and some osteopathic physicians. Many believe that in addition to aligning the body, chiropractic adjustment balances the energy flow through the body in a way similar to the concept of qi that underlies many Asian medical therapies.

The word *chiropractic* comes from the Greek words *cheir,* meaning "hand," and *praktos,* meaning "done": "done by hand." The name was chosen by the developer of chiropractic, Daniel David Palmer, a Canadian who founded this healing discipline in the Midwestern United States in the 1890s. Palmer called it "a science of healing without drugs." Chiropractic's origins lie in the old folk medicine tradition of bonesetting, and as it evolved it incorporated principles of vitalism, spiritual inspiration, and rationalism. Most modern practitioners tend to incorporate scientific research into chiropractic, combining the materialistic reductionism of science with the metaphysics of their predecessors and the holistic paradigm of wellness.

Throughout its history, chiropractic has been controversial, and for almost its entire history, it has been at odds with the mainstream medical establishment. The American Medical Association called chiropractic an "unscientific cult" in 1966 and boycotted it until losing an antitrust lawsuit in 1987. The ruling judge stated that the AMA had engaged in an unlawful conspiracy "to contain and eliminate the chiropractic profession," and that it "had entered into a long history of illegal behavior."[1] Yet chiropractic has had a strong political base and sustained demand for services since its founding. In recent decades it has gained legitimacy and greater acceptance among medical doctors and health plans in the United States, and evidence-based medicine has been used to review research studies and generate practice guidelines.

Over 90 percent of people seen by chiropractors seek care for musculoskeletal pain, primarily back pain, neck pain, and headache. Chiropractors also treat painful extremity disorders, including sprain and strain injuries and carpal tunnel syndrome. A special review panel commissioned under a major grant received by the coauthor of this book, Marc Micozzi, with support from the U.S. Department of Health and Human Services, reviewed over seven hundred published research studies worldwide and determined that spinal manual therapy is the safest and most effective treatment for both acute and chronic back pain.[2]

HOW DOES IT WORK?

Chiropractors have historically emphasized the innate relationship in the body between structure and function, the mediating role of the nervous system, and the need for restoration and maintenance of structural and functional balance of the spine and musculoskeletal system. From this perspective, balance is key, and the presence or absence of pain is incidental. For patients, however, pain is almost always the primary concern. The public identifies chiropractors as musculoskeletal specialists, and the profession's reputation is largely based on chiropractors' ability to help people with their pain.

Chiropractors trace their healing roots to principles shared with other natural healing arts:

- Humans possess an innate self-healing potential, an "inner wisdom of the body."

- Accessing this self-healing system is the primary goal of the healing arts.
- Addressing the cause of an illness should take precedence over suppressing its symptoms.
- Drug suppression of symptoms can compromise and diminish the body's ability to heal itself; natural, nonpharmaceutical measures should generally be an approach of first resort, not last.
- A balanced, natural diet is crucial to good health.
- Regular exercise is essential to proper bodily function.

These principles, endorsed and elucidated by chiropractors since chiropractic was founded in the nineteenth century, are now widely recognized as the foundation of good health. Conventional medicine engages in symptom suppression and frequently assumes that the location of pain is also the site of its cause and origin. Thus, knee pain is generally assumed to be a knee problem, shoulder pain is assumed to be a shoulder problem, and so forth. This pain-centered diagnostic logic frequently leads to increasingly sophisticated and invasive diagnostic and medical procedures. For example, if physical examination of the knee fails to define the problem clearly, the knee is radiographed. If the X-ray fails to offer adequate clarification, magnetic resonance imaging (MRI) of the knee is performed, and in some cases a surgical procedure follows. All the while this search for knee pain may be missing the obvious fact that the pain is caused by misalignment of the hip at the pelvis. We should all remember that old spiritual "Dem Bones":

> *Knee bone connected to the thigh bone*
> *Thigh bone connected to the hip bone*
> *Hip bone connected to the back bone*
> *Back bone connected to the shoulder bone . . .*

Chiropractors also use diagnostic tools such as radiography and MRI. The point is not to disregard these new technologies, but to present an alternative diagnostic model. There are many people in pain for whom this entire high-tech diagnostic scenario gets played out, after which the poor person finally stumbles into the office of a chiropractor (if he or she can still walk), where the knee problem is discovered to be a compensation for a mechanical disorder in the low back, a common condition that too often remains outside conventional medicine's diagnostic loop. This person is fortunate if he or she found the chiropractor before surgery was scheduled. The reality is that when the low back is mechanically dysfunctional and in need of adjustment, this condition often places unusual stress on one or both knees. In such a case, medical doctors can and often do spend months or years medicating the knee symptoms or performing useless surgery, often failing to address the real source of the problem.

A WHOLE-BODY APPROACH

The chiropractic approach to musculoskeletal pain involves evaluating the pain in both a site-specific and whole-body context. These chiropractic principles reveal something unexpected: although chiropractic is best known for its success in the relief of musculoskeletal pain, it sometimes does not directly address pain relief. Instead, the practitioner focuses on the correction of structural and functional imbalances, which in some cases cause pain. Although shoulder, elbow, and wrist problems can be caused by injuries or pathologies in these areas, pain in and around each of the shoulder, elbow, and wrist joints can also have as its source segmental dysfunction—what is known as "subluxation"—in the cervical spine.

Subluxation is when one or more of the bones of your spine (the vertebrae) move out of position and create pressure on and irritation of the spinal nerves. Similarly, symptoms in the hip, knee, and ankle can also originate at the site of the pain, but in many cases the source lies in the lumbar spine or sacroiliac joints. Besides pain, other neurological symptoms such as tingling, tickling, pricking, or a sensation of burning can have a similar cause. The source of the pain should be sought along the path of the nerves leading to and from the site of the symptoms. Pain in the knee might come from the knee itself, but tracing the nerve pathways between the knee and the spine reveals possible areas of causation in and around the hip, in the deep muscles of the buttocks or pelvis, in the sacroiliac joints, or in the lumbar spine. If joint dysfunction does exist at the fourth and fifth lumbar levels, it might in turn have its primary source at L4 and L5, or it might represent a compensation for another subluxation elsewhere in the spine, perhaps above, in the lower or middle thoracic vertebrae, or below, in a mechanical dysfunction of the muscles and joints of the feet.

HOW BAD IS
YOUR LOW-BACK PAIN?

Low-back pain can be divided into acute, subacute, and chronic. While definitions vary, acute pain is commonly defined as having been present three weeks or less; subacute pain, between three weeks and three months; and chronic pain, longer than three months, or more than six episodes during twelve months. Long ago, after spinal manual therapy was proven effective in treating back pain, it was still being challenged by the medical establishment, which claimed it could work for acute but not for chronic pain (or vice versa). Accordingly, spinal manual therapy has now been proven to be effective for both of these types of back pain. Distinguishing between the two is important so that acute back pain can be prevented from becoming a chronic condition. Since low-back pain is the most common cause of pain and disability in working Americans, avoiding the development of chronic back pain out of acute back pain has become an important focus for chiropractic and other health care disciplines that deal with low-back pain.

Over five hundred studies on spinal manipulation for treatment of acute, subacute, and chronic low-back pain have been done. For example, a large study in Great Britain involving more than seven hundred patients compared spinal manipulation (a chiropractic technique) with standard hospital outpatient treatment for low-back pain, which consisted of physical therapy and wearing a corset. The study discovered that for patients with low-back pain in whom chiropractic manipulation is not contraindicated, chiropractic almost certainly confers worthwhile long-term benefits in comparison to hospital outpatient management.[3]

Acute versus Chronic Low-Back Pain

Strong agreement exists about the appropriateness of manipulation for many acute low-back pain cases, but debate still surrounds chronic low-back pain. For example, when one 1998 study rated the "appropriateness" of decisions to initiate manipulative therapy, it was deemed that manipulation was "inappropriate" for chronic low-back pain. Although this rating lowered the percentage of cases for which chiropractic was considered appropriate, this study's researchers aptly noted that the study still offered solid justification for primary-care physicians to refer many more of their low-back pain patients to chiropractors.[4]

A more systematic review on manual therapies for low-back and neck pain, undertaken in 2004, concluded that spinal manipulation has demonstrated effectiveness for patients with low-back pain, whether categorized as acute, chronic, or combined acute and chronic.[5] Because the prognosis for patients with acute low-back pain is better than for those with chronic pain, high priority should be given to preventing acute cases from becoming chronic. Conventional medicine says that 90 percent of low-back pain resolves on its own within a short time. However, findings published in 1995 in the *British Medical Journal* seriously question the assumption that most low-back pain patients seen by primary-care physicians get resolution of their complaints.[6] And a 1998 study found that at three-month and twelve-month follow-ups, only 21 percent and 25 percent, respectively, had completely recovered in terms of pain and disability, and only 8 percent of patients continued to consult their physician for longer than three months.[7] In other words, the oft-quoted 90 percent figure in reality applies to the number of patients who give up on getting resolution of their problem from their physicians, not the number who stop seeing their doctors because they recovered from their back pain.

We should stop characterizing low-back pain in terms of a multitude of acute problems, most of which get better, and a small number of chronic long-term problems. Low-back pain should be viewed as a chronic problem with a messy pattern of complaining symptoms and periods of relative freedom from pain and disability, interspersed with acute episodes, exacerbations, and recurrences. There are two consistent observations about low-back pain: (1) having had a previous episode of low-back pain is the strongest predictor for having a new episode (past behavior is the best predictor of future behavior); and (2) by the age of thirty almost half the population will have experienced a substantial episode of low-back pain. These facts simply do not fit with claims that most episodes of low-back pain end in complete recovery. The people in the aforementioned 1998 British study were not referred for manual manipulation, and most then went on to develop chronic low-back pain. Based on current guidelines, which emphasize the functionally restorative qualities of chiropractic manipulation, it is reasonable to conclude that early chiropractic adjustments can prevent the progression of an acute problem to a chronic problem in many people.

So, how acute is your back pain? To someone suffering with back pain, the conclusion is simple: seek chiropractic—the sooner the better, if you want to avoid a chronic problem.

THE PROVEN EFFECTIVENESS OF CHIROPRACTIC

If statistics are one measure of the benefits of chiropractic for a number of problems, consider the following: Use of chiropractic in the United States tripled between 1980 and 2000, from about 4 percent to an estimated 12 percent of the population.[8] American chiropractors log approximately 190 million patient visits per year, or about 30 percent of visits to all CAM practitioners, representing a nearly $30 billion industry in the United States alone.[9] In recent years, the mainstreaming of chiropractic has taken many forms. Government agencies in the United States, Great Britain, Australia, New Zealand, Denmark, and Sweden have recognized spinal manipulation as one of a very small number of effective treatment methods for low-back pain, the condition most often treated by chiropractors—and the most common cause of pain and disability in working-age Americans. U.S. guidelines established by the Department of Health and Human Services found that only two categories of professionally administered procedures (spinal manipulation and anti-inflammatory or analgesic medications) had proven effective for this widespread problem, and that only manipulation provided both pain relief and functional improvement.

Back Pain

While it may seem counterintuitive, one of the most important and simplest things you can do when your lower back is sore is to keep moving! Gentle exercise such as walking and swimming are good for your lower back, provided you have not developed a disabling condition. In fact, not moving enough contributes to developing the discomfort in the first place. Walking can be as effective as clinic-run rehabilitation programs for back pain, and it only takes as little as twenty minutes twice a week.

Acupuncture, which we'll look at in chapter 10, is another effective way to relieve low-back pain. No less an authority than Sir William Osler (1849–1919), the "Father of Modern Medicine," a Canadian physician and one of the four founding professors of the Johns Hopkins University Hospital, recommended acupuncture for the treatment of "lumbago," or low-back pain, in the 1910 edition of his classic textbook of medicine, *The Principles and Practice of Medicine*. Unfortunately, and perhaps unsurprisingly, all mention of acupuncture disappeared in subsequent editions of his textbook published after his death.

But the number one, proven treatment for relieving back pain and restoring function, based on decades of scientific data, is indisputably spinal manual therapy—a chiropractic adjustment. In a 2003 investigation of 115 patients with chronic spinal pain, researchers compared the effects of medication, spinal manipulation, and acupuncture. The highest proportion of early recovery was found for manipulation (30 percent), followed by acupuncture (10 percent), and finally medication (5 percent). Manipulation also outperformed the other interventions on a variety of other measures, with one notable exception:

acupuncture achieved the best results on the visual analog scale for neck pain improvement.[10]

In 2009, the first randomized controlled trial of chiropractic care for older adults was undertaken—one of the first studies to compare different methods of chiropractic adjustment to one another and to standard medical care.[11] Researchers evaluated the effects of these different approaches in 240 people with subacute and chronic low-back pain. Both "high-velocity" and "low-velocity" adjustment techniques (relating to how quickly the adjustment is performed) resulted in similar levels of improvement, with both chiropractic methods substantially outperforming the medical care group, which also received the same exercise instructions as the chiropractic groups, only with the addition of pain medication.

In another study, a team at the National Spine Center in Canada looked at guidelines-based care (including chiropractic spinal manipulation) versus standard care by family-practice physicians for acute low-back pain of sixteen weeks or less in duration. The researchers found that guidelines-based chiropractic care was significantly more effective. They also found, not surprisingly, that typically medical doctors did not abide with guidelines, with 78 percent of patients receiving prescriptions for dangerous narcotic drugs (e.g., Tylenol 3, a liver toxin containing codeine) that were not guidelines-endorsed.[12] The results of this study so alarmed the editors of *Spine Journal*, a peer-reviewed medical journal, that they implored doctors to adhere more closely to evidence-based guidelines with regard to ordering fewer prescriptions for narcotic opioid drugs for patients and including more proven mind-body modalities.

Low-Back Pain with Leg Pain

Appropriate care is important for those in whom low-back pain radiates into the leg. In such cases, testing is appropriate to screen for signs of radiculopathy, where the problem occurs at or near the root of the sciatic nerve, shortly after its exit from the spinal cord, or for signs of cauda equina syndrome, a serious neurologic condition in which damage to nerve bundles of the spine causes loss of function. However, one

British study of primary-care practitioners found that a majority of these physicians did not routinely examine for muscle weakness or sensations, and nearly one-third did not regularly check reflexes.[13] Given increasing limitations on the time doctors can spend examining patients and increasing reliance on blood tests and other kinds of testing without doing physical examinations, this situation has probably only gotten worse. Currently, U.S. Department of Health and Human Services guidelines state that spinal manipulation is appropriate for acute low-back pain that includes nonradicular pain radiating into the leg. In cases where radicular signs, such as muscle weakness or decreased reflex response, are present, there is still some evidence to suggest that chiropractic can yield benefit.

Carpal Tunnel Syndrome
In the chiropractic field over the past decade, the arms and legs have become increasingly recognized as being responsive to manual therapy. Compression of the median nerve at the wrist can lead to carpal tunnel syndrome, involving painful feelings in the fingers, with or without pain in the wrist, palm, and/or forearm above the area of compression. One of its major causes is protracted strain on an extended or flexed wrist caused by repetitive stress—a situation found in many workplaces. Manipulation takes pressure off the transverse carpal ligament and added wrist adjustments help decompress the carpal tunnel. Studies on chiropractic intervention in the management of carpal tunnel syndrome suggest that a broad array of dietary, exercise, and manipulative interventions results in significant improvements in strength and improved pain and distress for at least six months post-treatment.[14] Chiropractic manipulation can yield improvement in situations where shoulder pain is involved, although corticosteroid injections produced more rapid improvements.[15]

Headache
Headache is a condition for which manual adjustment, usually of the cervical spine, has been found to be effective. The International Headache Society classifies benign headaches into three major

groups—tension-type, cervical (from the neck), and migraine. While a headache from any category can be quite painful, migraines are generally the most severe and disabling, while tension-type headaches are the mildest.

Tension-Type Headache

A study conducted at Northwestern College of Chiropractic in Minnesota found chiropractic to be more effective than the prescription medication amitriptyline for long-term relief of tension-type headache pain.[16] Further, chiropractic patients maintained their levels of improvement after treatment was discontinued, whereas those taking medication returned to pretreatment status on the average of one month after discontinuation. This example demonstrates that while medications suppress symptoms, chiropractic addresses the problem at a more causal level. Chiropractic treatment of tension headaches is supported by other clinical studies as well.

Migraine and Other Types of Headaches

Using a similar approach in the chiropractic treatment of migraine headaches, another study conducted at Northwestern College of Chiropractic observed comparable results to what was found in the aforementioned tension-type headache study and determined that there was no advantage to combining amitriptyline along with spinal adjustment for treatment.[17] Another later study reported improvements from manipulation in migraine headache frequency, duration, disability, and level of medication.[18]

In an investigation of one hundred patients with chronic migraine headaches treated by manipulation, an absence of headaches was reported in one-quarter of participants and an improvement in over one-third of the patients six months after completing treatment, while the remaining third reported improvement that lasted for approximately one month.[19] Comparing cold-pack treatment with mobilization, another study showed a reduction of post-traumatic headache pain by nearly 50 percent with spinal manual therapy compared to cold therapy after two weeks.[20]

Other Headache Approaches

The U.S. Department of Health and Human Services' Agency for Healthcare Research and Quality started a review of the literature on headaches as part of its ongoing process of guidelines development (which included the low-back guidelines discussed earlier in this chapter). However, after complaints from surgeons about their findings that spinal therapy is preferable to surgery for low-back pain, Congress cut funding to the agency, which eliminated all future guidelines development and stopped work on all pending guidelines. The agency's committee, which had been performing the evaluation and developing ratings based on the evidence, was ultimately sent to the Duke University Center for Health Policy Research and Education, which later produced a report based on the work begun by the agency.[21]

Among the physical interventions reviewed in this report were cervical spinal manipulation, cranial-sacral therapy, massage (including trigger-point release), mobilization, stretching, heat therapy, ultrasound, transcutaneous electrical nerve stimulation, surgery, and exercise. Among the behavioral interventions reviewed were relaxation, biofeedback, cognitive-behavioral (stress management) therapy, and hypnosis. The final report concluded that nondrug treatments (including spinal manual manipulation) are of growing importance and may be the first choice for most patients.

Menstrual Pain

Two studies on chiropractic adjustment/manipulation for primary dysmenorrhea showed encouraging results for both pain relief and changes in certain prostaglandin hormones. The patients reported less pain in the abdomen and lower back.[22] Dysmenorrhea may be another condition for which chiropractic manipulation may help certain people.

Middle-Ear Infection

It is historically noteworthy that the first spinal manual adjustment by D. D. Palmer in the 1890s resulted in the restoration of hearing to a deaf janitor, Harvey Lillard. In more recent times, J. M. Fallon, a New York pediatric chiropractor, evaluated chiropractic treatment for children with otitis media, or middle-ear infection. Taking into consideration both parental reports and studies of the eardrums of more than four hundred patients, results demonstrated improved outcomes compared to waiting out the natural course of the illness. This research data suggests a positive role for spinal and cranial manipulation in the management of this common condition in children, where in many cases the intensive use of antibiotics can be quite challenging, counterproductive, and even dangerous to the child.[23]

Neck Pain

Chiropractors have treated chronic and acute neck pain and related upper-extremity symptoms since the profession's beginnings. A 2007 review of the literature analyzed sixteen trials on manual therapies for chronic neck pain not due to whiplash (nine for manipulation, five for mobilization, and two for other manual methods). The investigators found evidence that subjects with chronic neck pain not due to whiplash and without arm pain and headache showed clinically important improvements from a course of spinal manipulation or mobilization at 6 weeks, at 12 weeks, and up to 104 weeks post-treatment. They also found that current evidence does not support a similar level of benefit for the same conditions from massage.[24]

Surgery: Before and After

Chiropractic uses neither drugs nor surgery. However, many people who are possible surgical candidates consult chiropractors as their initial point of contact with the health care system. Thus an important aspect of the chiropractor's role is to evaluate painful conditions that may ultimately require surgery. To properly serve their patients, many chiropractors develop working relationships with neurosurgeons and orthopedic surgeons in their communities—for example, in the modern "spine center." In some cases, if the chiropractic examination reveals major abnormalities of motor, reflex, or sensory nerve function indicative of cauda equina syndrome or severe nerve-root compression, referral to a surgeon may be immediate. In less severe cases a trial of chiropractic care is attempted for up to a month. If this approach fails to result in significant improvement, surgical referral often follows.

Chiropractors also sometimes provide ongoing treatment in cases where surgery has not helped or has even harmed the patient. While the specific site of a healed surgical procedure should not be directly treated, it is common for adjacent areas (e.g., the sacroiliac joints) to require adjustment after a surgical site has healed. Such manual manipulation often provides significant pain relief.

BOUNDARY TYPES: WHO BENEFITS AND WHY

Chiropractic is a form of manual therapy—working with the body to influence the health of the body and mind—so its relationship to boundaries is similar to that of bodywork and massage, with some distinctions.

Your visit to the chiropractor is more like a visit to a doctor. Your visit will be shorter, and less intimate, than with a massage therapist, and you won't have to take your clothes off. The therapy is more procedural, with specialized equipment and techniques, as well as clinical protocols. It moves beyond your boundaries, your body, and the simple touch and contact of the massage therapist. For correcting imbalances in the skeleton that influence body and mind, chiropractic is well studied by research and there are no clear distinctions that it works for one boundary type or the other.

A thick boundary person may be comfortable with a chiropractic session for the reasons reviewed above, since it does not cross or challenge physical boundaries as much compared to getting a massage. Chiropractic adjustment should also work well for those with thick boundaries because it leaves no doubt that the practitioner is really "doing something" to the body, as there will be physical sensations, movements, and sounds associated with the adjustment.

Different styles of chiropractic, such as high-velocity, are more vigorous than others, such as low-velocity, and may be adjusted by the practitioner as suited to the comfort zone of your boundary type.

FINDING A PRACTITIONER

There are nearly one hundred thousand chiropractors worldwide; two-thirds are in the United States. Chiropractors are now licensed throughout the English-speaking world and in an increasing number of other nations. Rigorous educational standards are supervised by government-recognized accrediting agencies, including, in the United States, the Council on Chiropractic Education. After fulfilling college science prerequisites equivalent to those required for admission to medical or osteopathic schools, chiropractic students must complete a four-year chiropractic school program, which includes a wide range of courses in anatomy, physiology, pathology, and diagnosis, as well as spinal adjusting, physical therapy, rehabilitation, and nutrition.

Chiropractic care is included in the U.S. Medicare system that serves the elderly and disabled. The majority of private health-insurance plans in the United States, including a majority of HMOs, include coverage for chiropractic services. Chiropractors serve on the U.S. Olympic medical staff, and professional sports teams across the country make chiropractic care available to their athletes. In the past decade, chiropractors have been hired as staff members for Veterans Administration hospitals and Department of Defense bases of all branches of the U.S. armed services. At the same time, chiropractors have attained staff privileges at hundreds of civilian hospitals, and there has been significant growth in the number of interdisciplinary and integrative clinics where chiropractors work alongside medical physicians and other conventional or CAM practitioners.

One of the best ways to find a qualified chiropractor is through another health care practitioner's referral or through a personal referral from a friend, as advice from someone with firsthand experience is always valuable when choosing any kind of health care practitioner. In addition, national associations such as the American Chiropractic Association and state chiropractic associations maintain listings of board-certified chiropractors.

If you have a specific concern or are seeking care for a child, for example, you may want to look for a chiropractor with specialization and experience in that area. Call the chiropractor's office and ask about the doctor's education and experience with particular pain conditions. If you have insurance coverage, you will also want investigate whether or not that specific chiropractor is covered under your plan. In general, chiropractic care is covered by most health care insurance plans in every state in the United States and by Medicare for defined conditions.

10

Acupuncture and Qigong

The practice of traditional Chinese medicine in the West, including the modalities of acupuncture and qigong, is exemplified by their use for safe and effective pain relief.

Acupuncture, or "sharp puncture," invokes impressions both simple and complex. The surface of the body, when compared in area with the point of the needle, provides an almost limitless number of locations in which the needle might be inserted. *Acupuncture* then becomes qualified in a variety of ways that appear to add meaning to the term but often obscure as much as clarify. Medical acupuncture, Western acupuncture, Chinese acupuncture, Japanese acupuncture, Korean acupuncture, Vietnamese acupuncture, new American acupuncture, Five Element acupuncture, traditional Chinese medicine (TCM) acupuncture, Taoist acupuncture, and classical Chinese acupuncture is a nonexhaustive (but exhausting nonetheless) list of some common types or styles of acupuncture represented in schools, workshops, publications, and scientific literature and on the Internet. In a new medical textbook on classical acupuncture therapeutics that Micozzi is working on with Kevin and Marnae Ergil, they are finding that none of these versions have available the complete tools that were developed over two thousand years in classical Chinese medicine to fully address all the problems in each person. There is much knowledge that remains to be restored to current usage. But the good news is that acupuncture is so powerful a technique that the wisdom of the body often responds to many different types and traditions of acupuncture.

Qiqong is an ancient Chinese health application that combines physical positions, breathing techniques, and focused intention, which are ultimately used as exercise and meditative practices. Qiqong, pronouned chee-kung, is the combination of two Chinese words that both mean the energy or life-force of the universe. Qiqong is a gentle exercise that anyone can perform.

The therapeutic modalities considered thus far in this book that are effective for pain come from historical traditions and modern research in the West. The subjects of this chapter, acupuncture and qigong, represent ancient therapeutic traditions from China that long anticipated the energy-mind-spirit connections described elsewhere in this book, principally by acknowledging the primary importance of a vital essence underlying physical functioning, called *qi* (or *chi*). The therapeutic goal of both acupuncture and qigong is to regulate qi.

ACUPUNCTURE COMES TO THE WEST

The medical use of acupuncture in Europe dates from the middle of the sixteenth century. Two physicians who traveled to Japan with the Dutch East India Company brought back their observations, and one of them, Willem ten Rhyne (1647–1690), a Dutch doctor and botanist, published *Dissertatio de Arthritide: Mantissa Schematica: de Acupunctura: et Orationes Tres,* on the art of needling, in 1683. In France, the Jesuit priest Jean-Baptiste Du Halde published a text in 1735 that included a detailed discussion of Chinese medicine that was based on returning missionaries' reports. In 1826, Franklin Bache (Benjamin Franklin's great-grandson) became one of the first American physicians to use acupuncture in his practice and printed the first account of this treatment in the United States (a fitting feat for the famous printer's descendant). Ten Rhyne's early text was in the library of the prominent physician Sir William Osler (1849–1919), who, in his *Principles and Practice of Medicine,* prescribed acupuncture for low-back pain. A century after Bache, French scholar and diplomat George Soulié de Morant published

L'acupuncture Chinoise, an extensive discussion of the practice of acupuncture based on direct translation, observation, and actual practice by the author. Published in 1939, the text was rooted in Morant's experiences in China from 1901 to 1917.

In England, James Morse Churchill, a member of the Royal College of Surgeons in London, published *A Description of Surgical Operations Peculiar to Japanese and Chinese* in 1825. Among early notable English acupuncturists were Dr. Felix Mann and Dr. Sidney Rose-Neil, both of whom began their explorations of acupuncture in the late 1950s and have influenced its development substantially in English-speaking countries.

Englishman J. R. Worsley, a physical therapist who began his studies of acupuncture in 1962, came to have a substantial impact on the perceptions of many practitioners in England and the United States. Worsley visited Hong Kong and Taiwan for a brief period and then became a part of the study group established by Rose-Neil. He went on to establish his Worsley Institute to disseminate his knowledge of Five-Element acupuncture to students of acupuncture in the West, including the United States.

Yet apart from the explorations of a few mainstream physicians with eclectic interests, the practices of traditional Chinese medicine remained the province of the Chinese communities in the United States in the middle of the nineteenth century. At that time, Chinese laborers arriving in America to seek work were accompanied by herbal merchants, entrepreneurs, and physicians. One of the most famous of these physicians was Doc Ing Hay, known as "the China Doctor of John Day, Oregon." Ah Fong Chuck, who came to the United States in 1866, became the first licensed practitioner of Chinese medicine in America when he received a medical license through legal action in Idaho in 1901. During the 1930s and '40s, stronger medical practice legislation, the interruption of the herb supply from China, and the advent of World War II made these practices disappear or retreat into the "Chinatowns" that had been established nationwide.

Then suddenly, in 1971, President Richard Nixon opened relations with China, and journalist James Reston's highly publicized appendectomy and postoperative care introduced the entire nation to the practice of acupuncture and Chinese medicine. Sudden visibility led to sustained public interest in the benefits of acupuncture and, gradually, to the licensing of practitioners and the development of training programs in many states. Today, most states and the District of Columbia license, certify, or register the practice of acupuncture and a range of other Chinese medicine activities, including the practice of herbal medicine by nonphysicians. There are at least forty programs in the United States that offer training in acupuncture and what is often called "Oriental medicine," an umbrella term that encompasses the medical traditions of China, Korean constitutional acupuncture, Japanese meridian therapy, and the interpretations of these traditions in the United States and Europe.

THE PRINCIPLE OF QI

When the vital energy known as "qi" and blood flow freely through the body, the person is in a state of health. When the flow of qi is interrupted by some cause—for example, an "evil" influence, a disturbed mental state, or trauma—illness results and pain can occur. The directionality of qi flow can be exploited by means of specialized needling techniques. To drain qi and so reduce activity in a certain channel, the needle can be oriented to resist the direction of the flow. To strengthen or supplement the qi in a channel or organ, the needle can be oriented in the direction of its natural flow.

The flow of qi is cyclical. During different parts of the day, as determined by ancient Chinese time-measuring methods of two-hour increments, the flow of qi will be strongest in one specific organ. This idea can be used in both diagnosis and treatment. In the course of one day the strength of qi will pass one time through each of the twelve channels. When the qi passes through a given channel, the organ associated with that channel is considered to be at its strongest. The qi of the organ associated with the channel on the opposite side of the "diurnal clock," or a specific time each day, is considered to be at its weakest. Thus, from 3:00 a.m. to 5:00 a.m., the qi of the lungs is at its strongest and the qi of the urinary bladder is at its weakest.

Clinically, this information may be applied in several ways. For example, if a patient consistently wakes up between 3:00 and 5:00 in the morning with an asthma attack, one might think that the qi of the lungs, which should be especially strong at this time, is instead exceptionally weak. Therefore, the person cannot breathe easily. In addition, other organs, such as the liver, take advantage of this weakness and overwhelm the lungs, causing an asthmatic attack.

As another example, if a person wakes between 5:00 and 7:00 in the morning with an immediate need to move the bowels, one might suspect that the qi of the large intestine (5:00 to 7:00 a.m.) is weak, and the qi of the kidneys (5:00 to 7:00 p.m.), which is responsible for securing the loss of substances from the body, is also weak and unable to restrain the large intestine.

Channels and Symptoms of Blocked Energy

Each of the channels has its own pathological symptoms and signs that guide the practitioner in determining a diagnosis and in choosing points for treatment. Pathology that is specific to the channel may present as pain, tension, rashes, and so on that manifest along a specific channel pathway. For example, a person with shoulder and arm pain that covers the posterior (backside) portion of the shoulder, then crosses over various muscles such as the scapular and trapezius muscle and goes down the posterior portion of the arm, might be diagnosed with stagnation of qi and blood in the small intestine channel, which causes pain.

Acupuncture and Pain

Pain is directly linked to an injury or to the interruption of the flow of qi. Acupuncture is employed to remove the obstruction and restore the flow. Needling may be used to remove the "evil" influence, to direct qi to places where it is insufficient, or to cause qi to flow where previously it had been blocked.

The ancient Chinese medical text *The Yellow Emperor's Classic of Medicine* described nine different needles for use in acupuncture. With the exception of one needle that appears to have had a specifically surgical application, the remaining eight needle types are still in use today, either in original or adapted form. Modern acupuncture also includes other tools and methods that have been added over the centuries.

One Western theory holds that acupuncture works by influencing endorphins, the body's natural painkillers. Solomon Snyder and Candace Pert's 1975 Nobel Prize–winning discovery of opiate neuropeptides—endorphins—helps us understand our perception of pain and, ultimately, pain control in people. The discovery of endorphins coincided with reemerging medical interest in acupuncture and acupuncture effects in pain control. By 1977, published studies suggested that some of acupuncture's effects in pain control (or "acupuncture analgesia") might be linked to the activity of endorphins. These studies showed that the effects of acupuncture analgesia, induced both by manual stimulation of acupuncture needles and by electrical stimulation, could be blocked by the administration of the opiate antagonist (blocker) drug naloxone.[1] This finding suggested that acupuncture's ability to control pain relies, at least in part, on its ability to trigger the release of endogenous opiates. Responding later to criticism that the reversal of acupuncture analgesia by the administration of naloxone was insufficient to validate the hypothesis that acupuncture analgesia was produced by endorphins, researchers provided a list of seventeen distinct lines of experimental evidence that support the acupuncture analgesia–endorphin hypothesis.[2]

HOW IS ACUPUNCTURE DONE?

The most common acupuncture tool is the filiform, or very fine metal needle, which can vary significantly in terms of structure, diameter, and length. A typical acupuncture needle has a body or shaft that is one inch long and a handle of approximately the same length. The distinctive part of an acupuncture needle is its tip, which is rounded and only moderately sharp, much like the tip of a pine needle. Solid and gently tapered, the acupuncture needle does not have the cutting edge of a hollow-point hypodermic needle. Its diameter typically is 0.25 mm ($\frac{1}{100}$ inch) or less. The insertion of an acupuncture needle is not painful, since it is so small and does not have a hollow point like the painful venipuncture needles used to draw blood by actually puncturing your skin and blood vessel.

Once the site for insertion has been determined, the needle is inserted rapidly through the skin and then adjusted to an appropriate depth. A twelfth-century classical Chinese text, *Ode of the Subtleties of Flow,* states, "Insert the needle with noble speed then proceed [to the appropriate depth] slowly; withdraw the needle with noble slowness, as haste will cause injury." Although a substantial number of considerations affect the angle and depth of insertion, methods of manipulation, and length of retention, the following description outlines a basic procedure. The essential aim is to obtain qi at the needling site, and the acupuncturist seeks either an objective or subjective indication that the qi has "arrived," known as "obtaining qi." The practitioner can sense the qi through his or her hands as the needle is manipulated or can determine its presence through observation of its effects or reports from the patient. The practitioner often feels the arrival of qi as a gentle grasping of the needle at the site, like a fish on the end of a line. The patient may sense the arrival of qi as itching, numbness, soreness, a swollen feeling, a local temperature change, or a distinct "electrical" sensation. Acupuncture points in different areas of the body respond differently, and these variations in response can be important diagnostic indicators. However, you should be aware that you might not necessarily feel any direct pain or responses from the needles. It is not unusual for a clinician to retain a needle in an acupuncture point where the qi has not arrived until the characteristic sensation occurs.

Once qi has been obtained, the clinician may choose to manipulate the needle to achieve a desired therapeutic effect. Methods range from simply putting the needle in place and leaving it there to engaging in complex manipulations that involve slow or rapid insertion of the needle to greater or shallower depths. These techniques may create a distinctive sensation along the channel pathway. The needle may be withdrawn promptly after qi arrives, or a short, fine needle (known as an "intradermal") may be retained in the site for several days. In all instances, the goal of the clinician is to influence the movement of qi.

One simple style of needle manipulation involves adjusting the direction of the needle to supplement or drain the qi at the particular channel point. If the acupuncture point is visualized as a hole where the channel qi can be touched and moved, this operation can either cause the qi to become secure and increase in the channel (supplementing) or cause the qi to spill out (draining).

Determining the Points

For the person who is experiencing the symptoms of "wind cold"—a Chinese term for a condition representing one of the "evils" that cause imbalance and disorder in the body and mind (it does not correlate to a specific Western diagnosis or pathology)—an acupuncturist might choose to needle a number of acupuncture points, including Wind Pool (Feng Chi, GB 20), located on the back of the neck below the occipital bone; Union Valley (He Gu, LI 4), located in the fleshy area between the base of the thumb and forefinger; and Broken Sequence (Lie Que, LU 7), on the forearm. These particular points could all be treated with a draining method, since in this case the channels are replete with the influences of the "external evils" of wind and cold. Wind Pool, as its name indicates, is often used to drain wind from the surface of the body, relieving headache and neck pain. Union Valley is an important acupuncture point that is used to influence the upper part of the body and to control pain. In this case, the point is used because of its ability to redirect wind, resolve the exterior, and treat headache and sore throat. Broken Sequence is said to dispel cold and to diffuse the lung. It affects the channels and can be used to treat sore throat and headache.

Another traditional Chinese method for choosing acupuncture points is based on their associations with what is known as the "five phases" or elements. Each of the phases corresponds to an organ: wood to liver, fire to heart, earth to spleen, metal to lungs, and water to kidney. Each phase is also related to a number of other categories, including taste, smell, climate, and time of day. If the person is displaying signs of vacuity of the water phase, a choice of points could be made from the transport points along the kidney channel associated with water, in order to supplement the water phase.

Points also may be chosen on the basis of the actual anatomic trajectory of the channel on which they lie. Union Valley is considered an important point for the head and face because the pathway of the large intestine channel on which it lies traverses that area of the body. Similarly, points on the lower extremities that lie on the urinary bladder channel, which traverses the entire back, frequently are used for back pain.

Finally, the practitioner often selects acupuncture points entirely on the basis of what he or she observes, and what you report, about their sensitivity to palpation, or on the basis of a variation in skin or subcutaneous tissue texture that the practitioner can perceive. Often, a number of acupuncture points in a specific area may be assessed to determine which would be most suitable for needling. In some cases, points that do not lie on specific channels or form part of the collection of recognized extra points may be identified by their tenderness. These points are known as *ah shi,* or "ouch, that's it" points, and they are an important part of clinical acupuncture's traditional history and contemporary practice.

With so many acupuncture points from which to choose and so many methods for choosing them, most practitioners focus on a few specific methods or a particular collection of points so they can develop expertise in the application of those key treatments.

Moxibustion

Moxibustion refers to the burning of dried and powdered leaves of *Artemisia vulgaris* (mugwort, or *ai ye*) on or near the skin in order to affect the movement of qi in the channel. *A. vulgaris* is said to be acrid and bitter and, when used as moxa, to have the ability to warm and enter channels. References to moxa appear in very early materials, such as the texts written on silk recovered from excavated tombs at Mawangdui, which date to 168 BCE.

Moxibustion can be applied to the body in many ways: directly, indirectly, by pole moxa, and by the warm needle method. Direct moxa involves burning a small amount of moxa, about the size of a grain of rice, directly on the skin. Depending on the desired effect, larger or smaller pieces of moxa may be used, and the moxa fluff can be allowed to burn all the way to the skin, actually causing a blister or a scar, or it can be removed before it has reached the skin. These techniques are used to stimulate acupuncture points where the action of moxibustion is traditionally indicated, or where warming the point seems to be the most appropriate response.

Indirect moxibustion involves the insertion of a substance between the moxa fluff and the patient's skin. This technique gives the practitioner greater control over the amount of heat applied to the person's body and offers increased protection from burning, allowing moxa treatments in such delicate areas as the face and back. Popular substances placed between moxa and the skin include ginger slices, garlic slices, and salt. The substance is often chosen because it has medicinal properties of its own that combine well with the properties of moxa. For instance, ginger might be selected in cases where vacuity cold is present, while garlic is considered useful for treating hot and toxic conditions.

During pole moxa, a cigar-shaped roll of moxa wrapped in paper is used to warm the acupuncture points gently without touching the skin. This method is a very safe application of moxibustion that can be taught to patients for self-application.

The warm needle method is accomplished by first inserting an acupuncture needle into the point and then placing moxa fluff on its handle. After the moxa is ignited, it burns gradually, imparting a sensation of gentle warmth to the acupuncture point and channel. This method is useful especially for people with arthritic joint pain.

QI CULTIVATION THROUGH QIGONG

Qigong, or qi cultivation, encompasses a broad range of practices and activities related to the meditative systems of Taoist and Buddhist practitioners, the health-giving exercises developed by ancient physicians, and the martial arts traditions of China. The common feature of these practices is the intention of enhancing qi by allowing the person to increase its quantity, smooth its flow, and place it under a greater degree of conscious control, thereby strengthening the body, mind, and spirit.

While Taoist and Buddhist qigong focuses on spiritual realization, medical qi cultivation addresses three areas: (1) self-cultivation, or the development of the practitioner's own health and stamina, (2) cultivation of the practitioner's ability to safely transmit qi to the patient, either by means of needles or directly through the hands, and (3) teaching patients to perform specific qigong practices that may address particular health issues or generally strengthen their qi.

HOW IS QIGONG DONE?

"Flowing water will never turn stale, the hinge of the door will never be eaten by worms," explains the *Spring and Autumn Annals,* a chronicle that has been one of the core Chinese classics since ancient times, attributed to Confucius. "They never rest in their activity: that's why."

Qi cultivation has been compared to flowing water. Ancient texts recovered at Mawangdui include illustrated guides to therapeutic properties and physical practices of a form of qigong known as "conduction" (*dao yin*). In the second century, a series of exercises were created based on movements of the tiger, deer, bear, monkey, and bird; these were practiced to ward off diseases. Zhang Zhongjing, an eminent Han dynasty physician, in his *Golden Cabinet Prescriptions,* recommends treating disease with dao yin and tui na, the exhalation and inhalation exercises fundamental to qigong.

Qigong has many forms of practice, which can be performed standing, sitting, or lying down. It always involves relaxation of the body, regulation of the breath, and calming of the mind. One form of qigong involves visualizing internal and external pathways of the channels and imagining qi moving along them in concert with the breath. As the practice develops, the practitioner begins to experience the sensation of qi traveling along the channel pathways. The mind guides qi to a specific area of the body, then the qi guides blood to that same area, improving circulation. This exercise is designed to train qi and blood to move freely along the channel pathways, leading to good health.

Another exercise involves the use of breath, visualization, and simple physical exercises to benefit the qi of the lungs. Assuming a relaxed posture, the practitioner begins by breathing naturally and allowing the mind to become calm. The upper and lower teeth are then clicked together gently thirty-six times. Saliva is produced, and it is retained in the mouth, swirled with the tongue, then swallowed in three parts. During this process the practitioner imagines it is flowing into the middle of the chest and then to an area about three finger-widths below the navel (one of three *dantian,* focal points for meditative and exercise techniques), corresponding to an important chakra in the ayurvedic system of medicine of India. At this point, the practitioner imagines that he or she is sitting in front of a reservoir of white qi, which enters the mouth on the inhalation and is transmitted through the body on the exhalation—first to the lungs, then to the lower dantian located near the navel, and finally out to the skin and body hair. This process of visualization is repeated eighteen times.

These exercises may sound odd, but they have been used for many centuries to enhance breathing, circulation, and other vital bodily functions, as well as to address the person's mental and spiritual state. The cultivation of qi is an integral part of traditional Chinese medicine, both within China and throughout the world.

THE PROVEN EFFECTIVENESS OF ACUPUNCTURE AND QIGONG

Together, acupuncture and its companion technique, moxibustion, are used to address a wide range of conditions and symptoms. Based on the simple premise that all disease involves disruption of the flow of qi, and that acupuncture and moxibustion regulate the movement of qi, there is, at least theoretically, no disease that cannot benefit from these methods. Scientific studies support the use of acupuncture for a wide range of pain-related conditions, including

- upper respiratory tract conditions
- acute sinusitis
- acute rhinitis

- common cold
- acute tonsillitis
- disorders of the mouth
- toothache, post-extraction pain
- gingivitis (inflammation of the gums)
- acute and chronic pharyngitis (sore throat)
- gastrointestinal disorders
- spasms of esophagus and cardia (junction of the esophagus and stomach)
- hiccups
- acute and chronic gastritis
- gastric hyperacidity
- chronic duodenal ulcer (for pain relief only)
- acute duodenal ulcer (without complications)
- acute and chronic colitis (irritable bowel)
- neurological and musculoskeletal disorders
- headache and migraine
- trigeminal neuralgia (shooting pains in the face)
- peripheral neuropathies (nerve disorders)
- intercostal neuralgia (pain between the ribs)
- cervical-brachial syndrome (disease of the neck and arm)
- sciatica
- low-back pain
- osteoarthritis

Substantial research efforts have taken place in Asia since the early twentieth century, and during the latter part of that century in the United States and Europe, and they are ongoing. Research approaches and standards vary widely and, like the practice of medicine itself, are subject to cultural influences. Where the West recognizes the randomized, placebo-controlled, double-blind clinical trial as the definitive standard for an "evidence-based" biomedical answer, other communities do not require or encourage their medical practitioners to secure knowledge or "truth" only in this highly artificial way. In addition, much of the research data that has been gathered is not accessible in the West due to language differences and difficulty of obtaining publications. As a result, the scientific communities of China, Japan, Europe, and the United States do not all have access to the same common sources of information and thus are not influenced by the same complete body of research.

Problems surrounding research design and methods have come to light as the Chinese medicine communities of the United States and Europe have conducted more research, and as the biomedical community as a whole has become better educated about Chinese medicine. In 1991, the U.S. Congress forced the National Institutes of Health to create the Office of Alternative Medicine (OAM), whose name has since been changed at least twice to suit the prevailing winds (currently it is known as the National Center for Complementary and Integrative Health). This center has hosted several conferences dealing with the issue of study design in the complementary and alternative medicine fields, including Chinese medicine. The center has also funded small research grants, some of which have been in the area of Chinese or Oriental medicine. Some of the studies being funded by the National Institutes of Health include:

- osteoarthritis (acupuncture)
- postoperative oral surgery pain (acupuncture)
- intractable reflex sympathetic dystrophy (acupuncture)
- muscular dystrophy (qigong)

In 1994, the NIH sponsored a workshop in cooperation with the U.S. Food and Drug Administration. Members of the acupuncture, allopathic medical, and Western scientific communities gave presentations detailing the safety and effectiveness of acupuncture needles. These presentations became the core of a petition that in 1996 led to the FDA reclassifying acupuncture needles from a class III experimental device to a class II medical device for use by qualified practitioners with special controls (sterility and single use). The coauthor of this book, Marc Micozzi, provided published references at the request of the FDA to facilitate this reclassification action.

In 1997, the National Institutes of Health convened a conference on acupuncture. For two days, experts in the field presented evidence on the safety and effectiveness of acupuncture in treating different specific medical conditions. The scientific panel that reviewed the presentations noted that acupuncture is widely practiced and studied in the United States, but much of the research was inconclusive due to problems in design, sample size, and other factors. The report concluded:

> Promising results have emerged, for example, showing efficacy of acupuncture in adult postoperative and chemotherapy nausea and vomiting and in postoperative dental pain. There are other situations such as addiction, stroke rehabilitation, headache, menstrual cramps, tennis elbow, fibromyalgia, myofascial pain, osteoarthritis, low back pain, carpal tunnel syndrome, gastrointestinal disease and asthma, in which acupuncture may be useful as an adjunct treatment or an acceptable alternative or be included in a comprehensive management program. Further research is likely to uncover additional areas where acupuncture interventions will be useful.[3]

And just two years earlier acupuncture needles had still been considered experimental!

Other organizations, such as the Society for Acupuncture Research (SAR), have emerged. SAR holds annual meetings and publishes its proceedings. Among its objectives are scholarly exchange between researchers in the area of acupuncture as well as other therapies related to Asian medicine, the encouragement of research activities by acupuncturists, and the clarification of research issues such as study design. In 1996, SAR compiled a summary of the most successful and well-designed clinical studies.

Researchers have been successful in obtaining measurable results when exploring such fundamental concepts as qi, the channels, acupuncture points, pulse diagnosis, and pattern diagnosis. However, these studies are difficult to design in ways that remain true to the traditional Chinese system, which is as much an art as a science, while obtaining data that will be recognized by the world's scientific community. For example, Chinese researchers, as well as researchers in the United States, Japan, and Korea, have been pursuing questions about the physiological basis of Chinese medical concepts like pulse patterns. This research typically includes applying pressure sensors over the radial artery, mimicking the way a clinical practitioner holds his or her fingers during a pulse reading. Pulse patterns are then recorded and correlated to determine the physical foundation of the diagnostic information the practitioner obtains from the pulse.

Research concerning channels and acupuncture meridians has relied on a variety of techniques, including the measurement of electrical resistance, thermography, tracing the pathways of injected radioisotopes, and anatomical dissection (although dissection has proved disappointing). Some notable work is being done to determine how the body's bioelectrical properties transmit information. The skin at many acupuncture points has a measurable lowered electrical resistance.

Even so, biomedical research may not be the right vehicle for understanding the fundamental principles of traditional Chinese medicine. It may be that the genius of Chinese medicine in these areas lies in its ability to generalize about the manifestations of incredibly complex biological phenomena in an articulate and clinically useful fashion. Clinical research studies have primarily been conducted in five areas: antiemesis (antivomiting) treatment, management of acute and chronic pain, substance-abuse treatment, treatment of paralysis due to stroke, and treatment of respiratory disease. Good clinical results were also shown in treatment of female infertility, breech presentation, menopause, depression, and urinary dysfunction.

Pain control is the most universal application of acupuncture, but it is also one of the most problematic areas to research. Some of the key problems in acupuncture research are: (1) Should the research investigator be trained in acupuncture? (2) Is acupuncture treatment appropriate for the condition? (3) Does the study allow for adjusting treatment to the individual patient's needs according to traditional diagnostics? (4) Are outcome measures clear? (5) Will placebo or sham acupuncture be used, and, if so, how will it be administered? (Unlike a prescription-drug placebo, how does one provide a control for the process of inserting a needle into the skin? Unlike herbal medicine studies, in which a placebo capsule can be administered, subjects in acupuncture studies always know whether they've been stuck with a needle.)

Despite these difficulties, effective studies can be cited. In one, acupuncture patients demonstrated a lower need for postoperative anesthesia following oral surgery than a group receiving sham acupuncture treatment.[4] Another study tracked forty-three women with menstrual pain; those receiving acupuncture experienced considerably less pain than the placebo and control groups.[5] When thirty migraine sufferers participated in a controlled trial, acupuncture was significantly effective in controlling the pain of their headaches.[6] A number of other studies demonstrated the effectiveness of acupuncture for back pain, lung disease, and sciatica. One study on back pain suggested that the use of acupuncture may produce a considerable cost benefit by completely eliminating the need for surgery.[7]

Like acupuncture research, the entire field of Chinese medicine presents inherent difficulties in designing effective studies. The cultivation of qi is highly personal and individualized, and it does not lend itself to standardized studies. However, a number of intriguing investigations have been conducted in China and, more recently, in the United States. Attempts to study the effects of externally transmitted qi have encountered problems with measurement. Some researchers believe qi involves measurable portions of the electromagnetic spectrum. Others theorize that qi exists but cannot be measured by currently available technology but only by observing its effects on the human body. Qi cultivation remains the challenging part of the broad fabric of China's traditional medicine.

BOUNDARY TYPES: WHO BENEFITS AND WHY

Thick boundary types tend to respond well to more hands-on approaches such as acupuncture because the intervention feels "real."

But acupuncture is also observed to work well for conditions across the boundary spectrum. At a more esoteric level—relating to energetic versus physical responses—those with thin boundaries sometimes report a sense of energy flow in their bodies that people with thicker boundaries are often unable to observe. The practices of acupuncture and qigong are particularly apt at creating this movement of energy.

Whether physical or energetic, thick or thin boundary, acupuncture offers a potent solution for your pain. When other options aren't right for you, you can almost always rely on acupuncture.

FINDING A PRACTITIONER

In China, acupuncture and other practices of its traditional medicine are mainstream medicine. Large hospitals entirely devoted to its practice offer acupuncture, herbal medicine, and tui na (see chapter 8) on both an inpatient and outpatient basis. It is not unusual to see a large outpatient facility treating twenty patients simultaneously in the same space. Smaller practices and even roadside stands also are common in China. Herbal prescriptions can be obtained from a Chinese herb store in almost any country that has a significant Chinese population. In Japan, small hospitals, large clinics, and private offices are typical settings.

Today, China's traditional medicine is practiced in various forms all over the world. It is truly a rare example of a global health system available worldwide, as is Western mainstream biomedicine (to those who can afford it). In some places it follows the contemporary patterns of traditional Chinese medicine. Elsewhere its practice is deeply influenced by local customs, preferences, or regional variations.

In office settings where Chinese medicine is practiced in the United States, the demands of record-keeping, insurance billing, biomedical screening processes, and clinic hygiene often produce a setting that looks very much like a typical physician's office, except for the presence of acupuncture needles, moxa fluff, and herbs.

Thirty years ago, few non-Asians had even heard of acupuncture or traditional Chinese medicine. Today, it is well known throughout the

ACADEMIC MEDICAL CENTERS OFFERING ACUPUNCTURE AND CHINESE MEDICINE

Center	Institution(s)	Location	Specialty	Research Areas in Chinese Medicine
Center for Addiction and Alternative Medicine Research	University of Minnesota Medical School & Hennepin County Medical Center	Minneapolis, MN	Addictions	Treatment of hepatitis C with Chinese herbal medicine, acupuncture, and relief of the symptoms of alcohol withdrawal
Complementary and Alternative Medicine Program at Stanford	Stanford University	Palo Alto, CA	Aging	Review of traditional Chinese medicine approaches to the problems of aging
Center for Alternative Medicine Research	Harvard Medical School	Boston, MA	General medical conditions	Acupuncture and back pain, acupuncture, and postoperative emesis (vomiting)
Center for Alternative Medicine Pain Research and Evaluation	University of Maryland School of Medicine	Baltimore, MD	Pain	Acupuncture and antiemesis, basic science research on acupuncture (animal model), acupuncture as an adjunct therapy for osteoarthritis of the knee, acupuncture for dental pain
Center for Research in Complementary and Alternative Medicine for Stroke and Neurological Disorders	Kessler Institute for Rehabilitation	West Orange, NJ	Stroke and neurological conditions	Ginkgo biloba in the treatment of stroke, qigong in the treatment of stroke, acupuncture in the treatment of dysphagia (difficulty swallowing) following stroke
Center for Complementary and Alternative Medicine Research in Women's Health	Columbia University	New York, NY	Traditional Chinese medicine in relation to women's health	Use of traditional Chinese herbal remedies for hot flashes

West and has become a staple of our cultural vocabulary. Initially opposed by the U.S. medical establishment, in recent years it has gained legal and professional acceptance. Interest, utilization, and acceptance has led to government funding for research at such respected academic institutions as Harvard and Stanford universities. While much about traditional Chinese medicine remains a mystery to many Westerners, it is clear that this ancient form of healing has moved into the world's medical mainstream, offering tremendous potential health benefits to the public for affordable, effective, and safe treatment of pain.

Although many health care professionals might use acupuncture techniques or claim to be certified in acupuncture, when seeking an acupuncturist or traditional Chinese medicine doctor it's important to work with someone who is licensed and who has advanced education and training. There are several ways you can find a qualified acupuncturist or doctor of Oriental medicine (DOM) in your area. One of the best ways is a referral by your physician or someone you know who has had personal experience with a good practitioner. There are also several organizations that can direct you to qualified practitioners in your area:

- The National Certification Commission for Acupuncture and Oriental Medicine has a registry of practitioners registered through that organization: www.nccaom.org.
- The American Academy of Medical Acupuncture has a directory of physicians who practice acupuncture at their website: www .medicalacupuncture.org.
- The American Association of Acupuncture and Oriental Medicine has a registry of practitioners listed by zip code: www .aaaomonline.org.

In addition to these referring organizations, there are a number of acupuncture and traditional Chinese medicine schools across the United States that provide low-cost acupuncture clinics where interns treat patients under the careful supervision of senior teaching staff.

This may be a viable option for many who want to integrate acupuncture into their regular health regimen and are on a budget, since acupuncture is typically not covered by health insurance plans—though acupuncture could save the health care system a fortune in expenditures on pain management, all without the hazards of pain drugs.

PART THREE

Managing Pain with Natural Products

The foregoing chapters have addressed how to work with the mind-body connection to influence the body through the mind, and the mind through the body, with benefits to both. Part 3 provides a presentation of the many natural constituents that can be introduced into the body through ingestion or inhalation that can have profound effects on mind and body for the management of pain.

11

Vitamins, Nutritional Foods, and Herbs

Vitamins, minerals, and herbal remedies are classified as dietary supplements in the United States, where their use has become commonplace. According to an industry survey, sales of just single herbal preparations in natural products stores are growing 5 percent a year, totaling tens of millions of dollars annually. Overall, sales of these preparations in natural foods, grocery, drug, and mass merchandise stores increased an average of 50 percent over the last decade.[1]

A 2000 telephone survey of over two thousand English-speaking adults shocked the medical world when it found that over 40 percent had used at least one alternative therapy, of which dietary supplement use was the most common form. In the same survey, nearly 20 percent of adults who regularly took prescription medication also reported the concurrent use of at least one herbal product or high-dose vitamin, and less than 40 percent of those surveyed who saw an alternative practitioner discussed their experience with their regular physician.[2] These findings are significant because interaction problems may arise when dietary supplements are combined with prescription or over-the-counter drugs, usually due to the more powerful effects of the drugs and their known and accepted side effects. The situation has only grown over time.

The pharmacological effects of dietary supplements are not surprising since many prescription drugs are derived from plants. For example, lidocaine and novocaine are derived from the coca plant (*Erythroxylum coca*), opioid pain relievers like morphine and codeine are derived from the seed pod of the poppy plant (*Papaver somniferum*), aspirin comes from meadowsweet (*Filipendula ulmaria*), digoxin comes from foxglove (*Digitalis lanata*), and warfarin is a derivative of dicoumarin found in sweet clover (*Melilotus officinalis*).

VITAMIN SUPPLEMENTS

The majority of herbal remedies and dietary supplements used in the United States today involves products that have therapeutic actions on the brain and central nervous system, including treatment of mood and pain. Studies indicate that vitamins, minerals, and other dietary supplements are safe and effective for the management of pain and several kinds of neurological problems. While individual vitamins and minerals can be obtained in supplement form, with some important exceptions (such as loss of magnesium and other minerals due to depletion of topsoil in which food is grown these days), they are also available in healthy foods, together with many other biologically active constituents that are not necessarily classified as vitamins. You can always try to find foods that contain the vitamins you need rather than relying on supplementation. But if you are among the 80 percent or more of Americans who can't or don't follow a healthy diet, it will be very difficult to achieve and maintain healthy vitamin and mineral levels without high-quality supplements (and not those gimmicky little once-per-day pills that purport to have everything you need).

B Vitamins:
Brain, Mind, and Nervous-System Health

We began this book discussing the effects of stress on health and the symptoms of disease like pain. When we are stressed, B vitamins are usually the first things that are used up by the body and the brain. B vitamins are responsible for your energy level on a daily basis, and stress exhausts a huge amount of energy. As well, deficiency in B vitamins is often caused from malabsorption during the course of aging. Deficiency can also occur from a poor diet, or due to autoimmune diseases, inflammatory bowel disease, and multiple sclerosis, conditions that interfere with the absorption of B vitamins from the gastrointestinal tract.

If you are taking Metformin to lower blood sugar, note that you should take a B vitamin supplement as this drug may interfere with absorption of vitamin B_{12}. Metformin is generally a safe and effective drug proven to manage diabetes and to prevent all the complications of diabetes in the eyes, heart, kidneys and peripheral nerves, including painful diabetic neuropathy. This "drug" is actually derived from French lilac (*Galega officinalis*), an ancient European folk remedy for sugar in the urine (diabetes mellitus). In the United States this herb is classified by the USDA as a noxious weed.

B vitamins are water-soluble nutrients found in many foods, primarily animal-based products such as red meat, poultry, eggs, fish, and dairy. The essential B vitamins include B_1 (thiamine), B_2 (riboflavin), B_3 (nicotinic acid), B_6 (pyridoxine), B_{12} (cobalamin), and folate (folic acid). These nutrients contribute to a wide array of physiological functions: red blood-cell production, nerve-cell function, metabolism of carbohydrates and fats, energy production, and immune-system function. They cannot be produced or stored by the body and therefore must be consumed through the diet or, especially if there is a deficiency due to any of the factors mentioned, through supplementation.

B vitamins play a significant role in protecting the nervous system and spinal cord, particularly B_{12}, which is critical for the fatty myelin tissues that protect nerve and brain cells. B vitamins along with other natural nutrients such as berberine, lutein, and choline can help maintain healthy brain function. In addition to affecting brain and nervous-system function, B vitamin deficiency, particularly B_{12}, can contribute to a sore tongue or mouth, weight loss, pale skin, weak immunity, rapid heart rate, diarrhea, menstrual dysfunction, burning foot pain, pernicious anemia, and even tumor development. Abnormalities in the stomach or small intestine can interfere with the biochemical intrinsic factor (IF), a glycoprotein produced by the parietal cells of the stomach that must bind with B_{12} for it to be absorbed in the small intestine, along with other nutrients.

A significant amount of data shows that B vitamins also play a role in cancer prevention. A 1999 study reported an association of low levels of B_{12} with breast cancer in postmenopausal women.[3] A 2013 study showed a protective effect of dietary folate against the development of colon cancer.[4]

Subclinical malnutrition may play a role in reduced cognitive function in some older persons. Folic acid deficiency, one of the most common nutritional deficiencies worldwide, has often been associated with cognitive disorders. In elderly patients the incidence of folic acid deficiency is particularly marked.

A study that evaluated nutritional status and cognitive function in men and women over sixty who had no known physical illnesses and were taking no medications showed that subjects with low blood levels of vitamins C or B_{12} had generally lower functions. Subjects with low levels of riboflavin or folic acid also had lower readings for some cognitive functions. These differences were significant.[5]

Interestingly, studies on vitamin B_6 and carpal tunnel syndrome show that it is useful as an adjunct treatment to conservative, nonsurgical therapy.[6]

Diabetic peripheral neuropathy is associated with vitamin B_1 (thiamine) deficiency. In a study in Tanzania comparing thiamine (25 mg a day) and pyridoxine (50 mg a day) therapy with placebo (containing 1 mg each of thiamine and pyridoxine), significant improvements in pain, numbness, tingling, and impairment of sensation in the legs were noted in the treatment group; the severity of signs of peripheral neuropathy decreased 50 percent in the treatment group compared to 11 percent in the placebo group.[7]

Riboflavin is a B vitamin and "neurovitamin" needed in the production of ATP as an energy source for all the cells in the body. Outright riboflavin deficiency is relatively rare in Western countries, but marginal deficiency (insufficiency) is relatively common, especially among older adults as well as some adolescents. A study of migraines found that 400 mg of riboflavin taken daily was superior to a placebo in reducing attack frequency and headache days. The dose of riboflavin used in this trial was quite high—about 300 times higher than the RDA.[8] However, riboflavin is quite safe and any excess is excreted in the urine, as is the case for most vitamins, with the exception of very few.

Vitamin C:
Blood Pressure, Joint Pain, Cancer

Recent research indicates that vitamin C may contribute significantly to lowering blood pressure as well as maintaining muscle mass and helping to prevent cancer. Researchers at the Johns Hopkins Medical Center found sufficient evidence from research studies that a 500 mg daily dose of vitamin C can lower blood pressure by five points. While it cannot take the place of blood-pressure medication, it may be a very useful supplement in the process of cutting back on the amount of medication one has to take (which is something you should always consult with a physician about to do safely).

With regard to muscle mass, the entire musculoskeletal system accounts for about 85 percent of the body's weight, mass, and size. Vitamin C is a collagen builder and extremely important for the regeneration of every cell in the body, and it supports bones and joints to reduce common joint pain. This nutrient is so important in so many ways that all animals make their own vitamin C except for two: humans and guinea pigs (one reason why guinea pigs originally became such an important laboratory model in scientific experiments). In fact, there has been more evidence on the potential health benefits of vitamin C than almost any other nutrient, as stated by Nobel prize–winning biochemist Linus Pauling, who promoted vitamin C for preventing everything from cancer to the common cold.

Vitamin D: Arthritis, Cancer,
Depression, Dementia, Diabetes, Multiple Sclerosis

Vitamin D has many critical metabolic functions. Knowledge of the role of vitamin D in metabolic activity and human health and identification of the forms and metabolic pathways for vitamin D had been building for many decades but has only become fully elucidated since the 1970s. Since then it has been discovered that vitamin D is actually recognized by every tissue in the body—every cell has receptors for vitamin D. It has been found to play a role in bone and skin health and blood pressure and may help in conditions as wide-ranging as cancer, diabetes, multiple sclerosis, and rheumatoid arthritis.

Vitamin D actually refers to a pair of biologically inactive precursors: vitamin D_3 (cholecalciferol) and vitamin D_2 (ergocalciferol). Vitamin D_3 is produced in the skin by a photoreaction on exposure to ultraviolet B light from the sun (wavelength 290 to 320 nm). Vitamin D_2 is produced in plants and enters the human diet through consumption of plant sources. Once present in the blood, both D_2 and D_3 enter the liver and kidneys, where they are hydroxylated to form both 25-hydroxyvitamin D and 1,25-dihydroxyvitamin D. The former, 25-hydroxyvitamin D, is relatively inactive and represents the storage form of vitamin D. By contrast, 1,25-dihydroxyvitamin D is highly active metabolically, and its levels are tightly controlled. Recently there has been some confusion in the literature regarding differences in the relative abundance, availability, and effects of vitamins D_2 and D_3, which have been reconciled by thoughtful investigation. The confusion centers on the fact that the major circulating form of vitamin D_3 in human blood is 25-hydroxyvitamin D_3, and therefore it is the form measured by physicians to evaluate vitamin D status in people worldwide. It takes a long time for this form to work on calcium absorption and mobilization, however, and it must be converted or metabolized to the more active 1,25-dihydroxyvitamin D for effectiveness in the body.

The first major functions of vitamin D to be recognized in scientific research were (1) enhancement of calcium absorption from the diet through the intestine and (2) mobilization and reabsorption of calcium from bone, which represents the major store of calcium (or "calcium bank") in the body. Calcium, in turn, is critical for cellular metabolism and membrane actions, enzymatic reactions, muscle function, skeletal structure, and a host of activities needed to sustain life and maintain homeostasis. Because vitamin D has long been recognized for its role in calcium metabolism, it has been used to treat patients with renal failure and bone diseases. It also has an important role in the treatment of postmenopausal osteoporosis and the current epidemic of bone fractures in the elderly. Vitamin D has also been used to treat hyperproliferative skin diseases such as psoriasis.

In the immune system, the large white blood cell macrophages activate vitamin D. The activated vitamin D in turn causes macrophages to make a peptide that specifically kills infective agents such as tuberculosis mycobacteria. Vitamin D also has a role in helping prevent autoimmune diseases such as multiple sclerosis, rheumatoid arthritis, and type 1 diabetes.

Vitamin D's activity in the kidneys has long been recognized, and it has been found to affect the production of renin and angiotensin, the major regulators of blood pressure, in the kidneys. There is a direct correlation between higher (further from the equator) latitudes (where both sunlight and vitamin D levels are lower) and higher blood pressure in both the northern and southern hemispheres of the earth. People at high latitudes who have high blood pressure experience a return to normal blood pressure levels after exposure to ultraviolet B light in a tanning bed three times a week for three months and restoration of active vitamin D levels. (And you thought it only worked if the sunlight was captured on a beach in the Bahamas!) Multiple sclerosis also shows a marked association with higher latitudes worldwide, and there may be a similar protective role for vitamin D for this disease.

Vitamin D is also thought to have an important role in the prevention of some cancers. As early as the 1940s it was noted that living at higher latitudes is associated with a higher incidence of several cancers (whereas only skin cancer specifically has a lower incidence at higher latitudes). Recent epidemiological observations have continued to bear out this association. A high frequency of sunbathing before age twenty was found to reduce the risk of non-Hodgkin's lymphoma. And, although sun exposure is related to an increased incidence of malignant melanoma, it was also found to be associated with increased survival from melanoma in a recent study.[9]

Low vitamin D levels are associated with low mood and higher rates of suicide and depression in studies at northerly latitudes worldwide.[10] The lack of sunshine associated with vitamin D deficiency is also associated with depression. Vitamin D is a fat-soluble vitamin, and inadequate intake of this nutrient may also be associated with inadequate dietary fat intake. All these problems have been compounded by faulty government recommendations to avoid dietary cholesterol and saturated fats. Unfortunately, there was never any evidence for any health benefits for a low-cholesterol, low-fat diet—and this dietary myth encourages well-meaning people to avoid eating healthy and delicious foods like butter, cheese, eggs, and meats, all of which are sources of protein and important essential fatty acids. When margarine substitutes for butter, for example, it leads to double the rates of chronic diseases.

Studies have shown the benefits of using vitamin D for dementia. The Institute of Medicine (IOM) originally recommended that adult men and women up to age seventy take in 600 IU of vitamin D daily based on a simple study over thirty years ago. And the recommended dietary allowance (RDA) for vitamin D for maintaining general good mental and physical health is 600 to 700 IU. But two recent studies, in 2014 and 2015, show that the calculations of the RDA for vitamin D are off by a factor of ten. Therefore, daily vitamin D intake should be 5,000 to 10,000 IU, accounting for the 1,000 to 2,000 IU that are generally obtained from the diet.[11]

Vitamin E:
Dementia, Diabetic Neuropathy

Recent studies compared high-dose vitamin E (2,000 IU) to a drug and to a placebo for treatment of dementia. Vitamin E showed remarkable benefits, while the drug showed no such effects. However, when the drug was given along with vitamin E, it negated the benefits of vitamin E alone.[12]

In a study of type 2 diabetes, vitamin E given for six months resulted in significant improvement in nerve conduction in the median motor nerve fibers in the treatment of diabetic neuropathy and pain.[13]

Iron: Restless Leg Syndrome

Iron deficiency, whether or not it results in anemia, appears to be an important factor in the development of restless leg syndrome (RLS) in older adults. In one study, patients with severe RLS had iron (as ferritin) levels of less than 50 mcg/ml. Lower ferritin levels correlated with greater severity of RLS symptoms and decreased sleep.[14] Lower levels of serum ferritin in RLS patients were also found in another study, and improvement in RLS symptoms was noted after iron repletion.[15]

It must be kept in mind that excess body iron stores—or iron overload—is associated with an increased risk of cancer and other chronic diseases, most likely related to the free radical–generating properties of unbound, free iron in the body, so caution must be exercised in dosing. Don't take iron supplements or supplements containing iron unless you have been diagnosed by your doctor with iron deficiency.

Lipoic Acid: Diabetic Neuropathy and Pain

Lipoic acid, also known as alpha-lipoic acid, appears to be promising in the treatment of diabetic neuropathy. In one study, patients with type 2 diabetes and symptomatic peripheral neuropathy were randomly selected to receive placebo or one of three different doses of intravenous alpha-lipoic acid (1,200, 600, or 100 mg) over three weeks. Total symptoms were significantly reduced in groups receiving 600 or 1,200 mg alpha-lipoic acid.[16]

Magnesium: Migraine Headache, PMS

Vitamins and minerals have been shown to be helpful for women for the related triple threat of migraine headache, premenstrual syndrome, and menstrual cramps. One of the most important supplements for women—and for anyone, for that matter—is magnesium, which is beneficial in both treating and preventing migraine attacks. Magnesium is essential for over three hundred biochemical reactions in the brain and body that use adenosine triphosphate (ATP). It is the fourth most prevalent cation, or positive ion (Na+, K+, Ca++, Mg++), in the body. After calcium (Ca++), it is the second most common divalent cation, i.e., carrying two positive charges (Mg++). However, dietary magnesium deficiency is quite common.

According to estimates of magnesium intake based on the third National Health and Nutrition Examination Survey (1988 to 1994), conducted by the U.S. Centers for Disease Control and Prevention, magnesium intake has been lower than the recommended daily allowance in both males and females between the ages of twelve and sixty in all racial and ethnic groups except non-Hispanic white males. The incidence of deficiency is even higher among hospitalized patients; 65 percent of those in intensive care, up to 12 percent of patients in general wards, and 30 percent of hospitalized alcoholics have low magnesium.[17]

Several studies indicate that magnesium supplementation may be helpful for the treatment of migraine as well as tension-type headaches.[18] Although the exact mechanism of magnesium's effects is unclear, it may interrupt the process at the vasoconstriction stage by interacting with serotonin and N-methyl-d-aspartate receptors, nitrous oxide synthesis and release, other migraine-related receptors, and neurotransmitters.

Excess magnesium causes diarrhea, an effect that was seen in every trial in which this data was collected. Inorganic forms of magnesium (magnesium oxide, magnesium chloride) may be more likely to cause diarrhea than organic forms (magnesium citrate, magnesium aspartate), but diarrhea can result from administration of any preparation. However, magnesium should not necessarily be avoided for this reason—in other words, a little diarrhea isn't all that bad for you when you consider the benefits. You don't want to let a little diarrhea discourage you from taking magnesium when you need it for pain.

In another study, adult migraine patients with an average attack frequency rate of four headaches a month received oral magnesium for twelve weeks to prevent migraine attacks. In the last four weeks, the headaches were reduced by nearly 50 percent. The number of days with migraine was also significantly decreased. Diarrhea was reported in 18 percent of participants, and gastric irritation in 4 percent of those receiving magnesium.[19]

Researchers have also long noted lower levels of magnesium in the red blood cells of women with premenstrual syndrome, with magnesium being an effective treatment.[20] Magnesium also reduces the need for pain medication.[21] In a study of menstrual migraines, women received 360 mg daily of magnesium pyrrolidine carboxylic acid or a placebo from the fifteenth day of their cycles until menses. Women receiving the magnesium had significantly less pain than the placebo group, and the number of days with headache decreased only in the magnesium group. The effects were so dramatic that for ethical reasons, after two months, the study was changed to an "open-label trial" in which magnesium was given to all patients for an additional two months. Significant decreases in pain were seen in both groups between the second and fourth months.[22]

There are also many studies on magnesium for other conditions mentioned elsewhere in this book, such as depression, arthritis, insomnia, and osteoporosis.

Zinc: Taste and Smell Disorders

Acute, severe zinc deficiency can cause decreased sensitivity of taste. Two studies found that taking 50 mg of elemental zinc a day significantly improved the sense of taste.[23] A study of over one hundred patients with loss of taste found that 100 mg zinc taken daily resulted in improvements. Zinc may be effective only in those with low serum zinc levels. Nearly one hundred patients in one study were divided into four groups, depending on the cause (zinc deficient, idiopathic, drug-induced, and other). All received zinc gluconate (22.6 mg twice per day) for four months. Zinc benefited the zinc-deficient and idiopathic groups but not the groups whose conditions were drug-induced or who fell into other categories.

In another study, patients with sensory-neural olfactory disorder were treated with usual drug therapy, zinc sulfate, or both. Of patients with post-traumatic olfactory disorder, those in the zinc sulfate groups had significantly greater improvements. For patients with disorders of postviral or unknown etiology, there were no significant differences in improvement among the three groups.[24]

Surgical and medical treatments for head and neck cancer often cause taste alterations. In a randomized, placebo-controlled study, patients receiving external radiation to the head and neck were randomly chosen to receive zinc sulfate (45 mg twice a day) or a placebo at the onset of taste alteration. The treatment was continued for one month after the radiation therapy had ended. Patients treated with placebo experienced a greater loss in taste acuity during radiation treatment compared to those treated with zinc. In addition, those treated with zinc had a faster recovery of taste acuity than those receiving placebo.[25]

COMMON
BENEFICIAL NUTRITIONAL FOODS

Scientists have long been aware that many fruits, vegetables, and legumes (beans) appear to reduce the risk of heart disease and cancer and help manage pain and other conditions. It has been hypothesized that these antidisease activities are present because these foods contain antioxidants (vitamins, minerals, and other constituents that protect cells from being damaged by oxidation). A larger group of disease-fighting nutrients is also being identified: phytochemicals, some of which are known commercially as "nutraceuticals."

Phytochemicals are thought to fight cancer and other ailments by keeping disease-causing substances from latching onto healthy cells and by removing toxins before they can cause harm. There are many thousands of phytochemicals—tomatoes alone contain ten thousand different kinds—each with slightly different functions. Genistein, for example, which is found in soybeans, prevents the formation of the capillaries needed to nourish tumors. Indoles, which increase immune function, are found in brassicas such as broccoli and cauliflower. The bioflavonoids found in limes and other citrus fruit prevent certain cancer-causing hormones from attaching to the body's cells. Much the way an earlier generation of scientists sought to identify and synthesize vitamins, today's researchers are working to isolate and prepare phytochemicals. However, it is unlikely that they will be able to reproduce the rich mix of beneficial substances found in a single tomato or a handful of veggies.

Bromelain: Irritable Bowel Syndrome

Bromelain, an enzyme derived from pineapple, is a potent source of digestive enzymes. A recent study found evidence that bromelain might have beneficial effects in the gastrointestinal tract for people with irritable bowel syndrome and may be clinically useful as an antidiarrheal drug.[26] A good serving of fresh pineapple or pineapple juice will provide bromelain in a food matrix together with other nutrients. Bromelain is also available as a supplement (many people cannot tolerate the high sugar of pineapple). There are many research studies on bromelain linking it to the treatment of various conditions and diseases. Athletes are increasingly taking bromelain to help manage sports injuries, and those undergoing surgery are using it to speed their recovery time. In addition, bromelain is being used in managing varied conditions such as sinusitis and inflammatory bowel disease and contains tumor-fighting properties.

Fiber: Crohn's Disease

Fiber is nondigestible complex carbohydrate, such as cellulose, present in any food of plant origin, including grains, fruits, and vegetables. It provides indigestible mass and matter in the GI tract that is important to GI function and motility and to eliminating food waste products from the body. There are many different kinds of fibers with varying effects on the GI tract in health and disease. Packaged cereal makers and their codependents at the American Heart Association and the National Institutes of Health present an oversimplified endorsement of "fiber" that does not wholly comport with the scientific evidence (or the lack of scientific evidence) about fiber. But the role and effects of dietary fiber are a complex issue under any circumstance.

Fiber is a particularly complex issue for people with painful Crohn's disease. If you've been diagnosed with Crohn's disease, whether or not you should eat high-fiber foods or take fiber supplements depends on your specific condition and where you are at any given point in the disease. In some people, fiber supplements like psyllium powder (such as Metamucil) or methylcellulose (such as Citrucel) may stop mild diarrhea. On the other hand, if your Crohn's disease has caused adhesions and strictures, high-fiber foods will cause pain and discomfort. Meanwhile, herbs that quell the chronic inflammation associated with Crohn's disease are slippery elm, cat's claw, and marshmallow plant (as a tea made from the herb, *Althaea officinalis*).

Fish Oil:
Depression, Multiple Sclerosis, Neuropathy

Omega-3 fatty acids are long-chain, polyunsaturated fatty acids (PUFAs) found in some plant and marine sources. These essential fatty acids, particularly docosahexaenoic acid (DHA), are necessary for cell membrane function and may be factors in depression, bipolar disorder, schizophrenia, and other mood and neurologic disorders. The Western diet contains considerably high amounts of omega-6 fatty acids but lesser amounts of omega-3 fatty acids—the opposite of what should be eaten for optimal health. Fish oil is high in PUFAs, DHA, and eicosapentaenoic acid. Nerve membranes contain high concentrations of DHA, as well as arachidonic acid (AA). Neurotransmitter receptors lie embedded in the nerve membranes, and their three-dimensional conformation is dependent on the fatty acids that give structure to the membranes.

Omega-3 fatty acids are key nutrients found in fatty fish varieties such as herring, salmon, bluefish, lake trout, and mackerel, and they are also available as supplements. Omega-3s have proven heart-health benefits, and they also have an anti-inflammatory effects (making them also helpful in treating irritable bowel syndrome). Omega-3s appear to work especially well for nerve pain. If you're going to supplement with fish oil, 1 to 2 grams per day is recommended. Biochemical studies have shown that high doses of omega-3 fatty acids lead to the incorporation of these compounds into the neuronal membrane phospholipids, which are crucial for cell signaling.

Omega-3 fatty acids are needed to insulate nerves so that they can send nervous impulses, or signals, effectively. An association between depression and multiple sclerosis is consistent with essential fatty acid depletion in both brain and nerve white matter and blood plasma. DHA is apparently absent in the adipose tissue of people with multiple sclerosis. Connections between abnormally low concentrations of omega-3 and high levels of omega-6 fatty acids and the occurrence of other neurologic disorders also have been noted.[27]

In one study, patients with neuropathic pain took large doses of omega-3 fatty acids daily. This varied from 2,400 to 7,200 mg/day of EPA-DHA. The patients suffered from nerve pain due to carpal tunnel syndrome, fibromyalgia, and other conditions. According to the results of the study, the patients experienced "clinically significant pain reduction" for up to nineteen months following the initial treatment.[28]

Garlic: Cardiovascular Disease, Cancer

Garlic has been widely promoted as a remedy for colds, coughs, flu, chronic bronchitis, whooping cough, ringworm, asthma, intestinal worms, and fever, as well as for digestive, gallbladder, and liver disorders. Investigators have explored its use as a treatment for mild hypertension (high blood pressure) and hyperlipidemia (elevated cholesterol), and it may have anticancer effects. Clinical studies of garlic in humans tend to address three areas: (1) effect on cardiovascular-related disease and risk factors such as lipid levels, blood pressure, glucose levels, atherosclerosis, and thrombosis; (2) protective associations with cancer; and (3) clinical adverse effects.

Scant data, primarily from case-control studies, suggests that dietary garlic consumption is associated with decreased risk of laryngeal, gastric, colorectal, and endometrial cancer and adenomatous colorectal polyps.[29] Cholesterol levels have been related to use of garlic as well.[30]

Currently, there is high consumer usage of garlic as a health supplement. Garlic preparations studied have included standardized dehydrated tablets, "aged garlic extract," oil macerates, distillates, raw garlic, and tablets with a combination of ingredients. Side effects of oral ingestion of garlic are garlicky breath and body odor. Other possible effects include flatulence (gas), esophageal and abdominal pain, small intestine obstruction, contact dermatitis, rhinitis, asthma, and bleeding. How frequently adverse effects occur with oral ingestion of garlic as a food, and whether they vary for particular garlic preparations, has not been established. Adverse effects of inhaled garlic dust include allergic reactions such as asthma, rhinitis, urticaria, angioedema, and anaphylaxis. Adverse effects of topical exposure to raw garlic include contact dermatitis, skin blisters, and ulcerative lesions. In particular, adverse effects related to bleeding and interactions with other drugs such as aspirin and anticoagulants warrant further study.

Ginger: Antinausea, General Pain Relief

Ginger, like garlic, can be considered to be both a popular ingredient in prepared foods and beverages and an effective medicinal plant remedy. Ginger has long been known and used for its antinausea effects and calming properties on the stomach; hence the traditional popular beverages ginger ale and ginger beer. It is particularly useful for nausea associated with pregnancy and with chemotherapy (for which acupuncture, as discussed in chapter 10, is also a useful alternative therapy). Ginger is also a useful pain reliever taken internally or applied topically.

Probiotics: Irritable Bowel Syndrome

Probiotics are a type of beneficial bacteria that are found naturally inside our intestines and aid in digestion. According to Dr. Joyce Frye, DO, "There is plausible rationale for why these would be helpful. If altered bacteria in the gut aren't the cause of the IBD (irritable bowel syndrome), it certainly is an effect."[31] Probiotics can be found in yogurts with active cultures and in sauerkraut and other fermented foods (kim chi, kombucha tea, etc.), or they may be taken in capsule form. But make sure you are taking a truly effective probiotic supplement.

Current research is constantly uncovering more aspects of the role of healthy probiotics in our GI tracts (called our "microbiome"), including brain functions that relate to pain perception, as well as specific potentially painful GI conditions.

HERBAL PAIN REMEDIES

Many safe, effective, and natural plant compounds help reduce chronic inflammation in the body and therefore help alleviate pain. In fact, many natural compounds appear to work like natural nonsteroidal anti-inflammatory drugs (NSAIDs), but without the dangers of those drugs. NSAIDs work by preventing the formation of certain prostaglandin hormones that cause pain, but their side effects have been so intense that one of them, Vioxx, was taken off the market in 2004 because of its toxic effects on the heart.

Ashwagandha: Joint Pain

Withania somnifera, also known as winter cherry or ashwagandha, is an ayurvedic remedy with potent anti-inflammatory and pain-relieving effects. As an adaptogen—an herb with homeostatic properties—ashwagandha seems to support overall health, allowing your body to better handle physical and mental stress. It is commonly used to treat back pain, as it nourishes muscle and bone tissues. It also has a relaxing effect on the central nervous system.

In 2004, Indian researchers conducted a thirty-two-week randomized, placebo-controlled clinical trial with participants experiencing chronic arthritic knee pain. They gave half the participants a standardized form of ashwagandha for thirty-two weeks, while the other half received a placebo. None of the patients in either group were allowed to take NSAIDs or steroids for pain relief.

At the conclusion of the study period, the ashwagandha group experienced "significantly superior" pain scores and very mild side effects.[32]

You can safely take up to 500 mg of ashwagandha root daily to relieve pain.

Boswellia: Osteoarthritis

Better known as frankincense, boswellia is an aromatic resin used in incense and perfumes, obtained from trees of the genus *Boswellia;* it is also a traditional ayurvedic remedy with potent anti-inflammatory and pain-relieving effects, especially for osteoarthritis.

In one investigation, researchers recruited thirty people with osteoarthritis of the knee. They randomly divided them into two groups. One group took boswellia extract for eight weeks, while the other group took a placebo. Then there was a washout period when both groups took nothing. After that, the groups crossed over and received the opposite treatment for the next eight weeks. All the participants—100 percent of them—reported decreases in knee pain when taking the boswellia extract. They also increased their knee flexibility and walking distance when taking the extract. The frequency of swelling in the knee joint decreased as well.[33]

When looking for any natural remedy for joints, make sure it includes an effective dose of boswellia. You safely can take 400 to 500 mg of it daily.

Capsaicin: Osteoarthritis, Rheumatoid Arthritis, Diabetic Neuropathy

Capsaicin is the active component in hot chili peppers and all plants belonging to the genus *Capsicum*. It also acts as an effective pain reliever. You generally find it in topical creams and ointments, but you can also take it orally—which you are doing every time you eat any variety of hot peppers. As a topical treatment, capsaicin depletes or interferes with a chemical called "substance P." This chemical transmits pain impulses to the brain, which makes capsaicin an ideal natural treatment option if you suffer from osteoarthritis, rheumatoid arthritis, and diabetic neuropathy.

In a 1991 study, patients with rheumatoid arthritis and osteoarthritis rubbed capsaicin cream or a placebo cream on their knees four times a day for four weeks. After just two weeks, 80 percent of those who used the capsaicin cream reported significant pain relief. The cream appeared to work slightly better for patients with rheumatoid arthritis compared to those with osteoarthritis.[34]

For pain relief, apply capsaicin three or four times a day. Rub the cream or gel into the painful area until it's no longer visible on the skin. You may experience a mild burning sensation, but it shouldn't be so strong that it's painful. Make sure you wash your hands thoroughly after applying capsaicin.

Ginkgo: Memory, Tinnitus, Vertigo

The ginkgo tree, *Ginkgo biloba,* is one of the oldest living species. The use of ginkgo has greatly increased since 1994, when Germany approved a standardized form of the leaf extract for the treatment of dementia. The standardized extract contains 22 to 27 percent flavonoid glycosides (including quercitin and kaempferol and their glycosides) and 5 to 7 percent terpene lactones (consisting of 2.8 to 3.4 percent ginkgolides A, B, and C and 2.6 to 3.3 percent bilobalide).

A 2010 study of over three hundred patients with Alzheimer's disease or multi-infarct dementia found that those who received *Ginkgo biloba* extract (120 mg/day) scored higher on the Alzheimer's Disease Assessment Scale cognitive subscale. After one year of treatment, nearly one-third of those receiving ginkgo showed improvement on the test compared with half that proportion of those receiving a placebo.[35] A 2003 six-month study of 216 patients with Alzheimer's disease or multi-infarct dementia found that those who were given 240 mg/day of a standardized ginkgo extract had significant improvements in memory, attention, psychopathology, and behavior.[36] In a 1996 study of forty Alzheimer's patients, those given 240 mg/day of standardized ginkgo extract for three months showed significant improvements in memory, attention, and psychopathology after just one month.[37]

Ginkgo may also have beneficial effects on memory impairment that is not related to Alzheimer's disease. In one double-blind study, thirty-one outpatients over the age of fifty who had mild to moderate memory impairment were given 120 mg of ginkgo a day. Researchers noted a beneficial effect with this therapy after twelve and fourteen weeks.[38]

A recent analysis summarized all published studies in which ginkgo was given for dementia. The patients were sufficiently characterized with a diagnosis of Alzheimer's disease or there was enough clinical detail for researchers to assign this diagnosis. The trials excluded those with depression or other neurological disease and excluded the use of other central nervous system medications. Researchers included studies that used standardized ginkgo extract at any dose, had at least one outcome measure that was an objective assessment of cognitive function, and contained sufficient statistical information for analysis. Although more than fifty articles were identified, the majority did not meet inclusion criteria in this meta-analysis because of a lack of clear diagnoses of dementia and Alzheimer's. Of the four studies that met all inclusion criteria, these involved 212 subjects in each of the placebo and ginkgo treatment groups. The authors concluded that three to six months of treatment with 120 to 240 mg of ginkgo has a small but significant effect on objective measures of cognition in patients with Alzheimer's disease.[39]

Ginkgo also appears to be a promising remedy for people who experience ringing in the ears and sudden hearing loss. Ten ear, nose, and throat specialists conducted a study involving over a hundred patients with tinnitus over a three-month treatment period. Patients were comparable in regard to duration and intensity of symptoms and degree of impairment. A significantly greater percentage of the ginkgo-treated group experienced either resolution of their symptoms or distinct improvement, regardless of the duration of symptoms, whether the tinnitus was bilateral or unilateral, and whether symptoms were constant or intermittent.[40]

In a therapeutic trial of acute deafness, *Ginkgo biloba* extract (320 mg/day) was given to one group of subjects and a standard drug, the alpha-blocker nicergoline, was given to the other group. The rationale for the design of this study was that a lack of blood flow may underlie acute deafness, regardless of the triggering event. From the tenth day until the end of the trial, improvement appeared to be greater in the ginkgo group, although both groups improved. The gain in the ginkgo group ranged between six and fifteen decibels greater than in the nicergoline drug group.[41]

In a comparison study on eighty patients with sudden hearing loss (of no more than ten days' duration), a ginkgo extract (175 mg intravenous infusion plus 160 mg oral/day) was compared with the standard drug used for this condition, a vasodilating, antiserotonergic drug, naftidrofuryl. After one week of observation, 40 percent of those in each group showed a complete remission of hearing loss, consistent with expected rates of spontaneous recovery. After two and three weeks of observation, there was no difference between the groups in relative hearing gain. Yet there was a borderline benefit of ginkgo over naftidrofuryl because no side effects were attributed to ginkgo, while some patients in the naftidrofuryl drug group developed blood-pressure changes, headache, or sleep disturbances.[42]

In a study on vertigo conducted over a three-month period, subjects received either 160 mg/day standard *Ginkgo biloba* extract or a placebo. The effectiveness of the ginkgo extract on the intensity, frequency, and duration of vertigo was statistically and clinically significant by the end of the first month. After three months, nearly 50 percent of the ginkgo-treated participants were asymptomatic, compared with less than 20 percent of those who received a placebo.[43]

Kava: Anxiety, Cancer

Piper methysticum, known as kava or kava-kava, is a psychoactive member of the pepper family originating in the western Pacific. Traditionally, the root of the kava plant has been used widely in Polynesia, Micronesia, and Melanesia as a ceremonial tranquilizing beverage. Kava has also long been used in Hawaii, Fiji, Samoa, Vanuatu, and other Pacific nations as an effective anti-anxiety agent. It is also now used medicinally in Europe and the United States for anxiety and insomnia and is approved and registered in Germany for the treatment of "states of nervous anxiety, tension, and agitation" in doses of 60 to 120 mg of kavalactones for up to three months. And now, new research shows kava's amazing ability to help prevent cancer.

In two studies, patients with various diagnosed anxiety and neurotic disorders received 70 mg of kavalactones three times daily for four weeks. The kava group demonstrated a significant reduction in anxiety.[44] In another study, 101 outpatients with diagnosed anxiety disorders (agoraphobia, specific phobia, generalized anxiety disorder, or adjustment disorder with anxiety) were treated with a kava extract for twenty-four weeks. The results showed significant reductions in anxiety.[45] In a placebo-controlled trial, fifty-eight patients with anxiety received 210 mg of kava or a placebo daily for one month. Compared with those receiving placebo, those receiving kava had significantly greater reductions in Hamilton Anxiety Scale (HAMA) scores, with improvements beginning within one week.[46]

About ten years ago, there was a false scare about the possible liver toxicity of kava. However, a study showed there was no real evidence pointing to kava for liver toxicity; researchers found that prescription-drug use was the likely culprit in the cases of liver toxicity that were observed.[47]

A new study has shown the potentially powerful ability of kava to prevent lung cancer. In fact, the study showed that kava reduced the formation of lung adenomas in mice (which are comparable to human lung adenocarcinomas) by 99 percent—an unprecedented prevention rate in studies using chemopreventive agents. The mice were subjected to tobacco carcinogen treatment and given a kava-derived dietary supplement on a daily basis. Compared to a control group, the kava group showed a 99 percent reduced rate of tumor growth; in fact, some of the mice given kava developed no tumors at all. And the type of DNA changes typically associated with heavy tobacco use were also significantly reduced, with no negative effects on the liver.[48] This lab evidence supports the observation that people living in the South Pacific, where kava consumption is common, despite tobacco use, have dramatically lower rates of lung cancer. In Fiji, the rate of lung cancer is only 5 to 10 percent of the U.S. lung cancer rate. That's a ten- to twenty-fold reduction in the lung cancer rate! That means that kava can reduce the risk of lung cancer as much or more than cigarette smoking is said to increase it.

A University of Minnesota research team is currently pursuing development of kava-derived drugs that may aid in both the prevention and treatment of lung and other types of cancer. A new patent-pending kava supplement enriched with cancer-preventive extracts is also planned to be used in human clinical trials.

Resveratrol: Postsurgical Pain

Resveratrol is a stilbenoid, naturally produced by several plants in response to injury or attack by pathogens. Resveratrol is a prominent constituent of red wine, as it is found in the skin of grapes. It also appears to block the body's pain receptors.

Researchers from the University of Arizona School of Medicine recently published a study on resveratrol in the medical journal *Molecular Pain*. They found that resveratrol "profoundly" inhibits two important pathways involved in the sensitization of peripheral pain receptors.[49] Plus, resveratrol may one day help you recover more quickly from surgery by inhibiting pain receptors.

In the United States, doctors perform more than forty-five million surgeries annually, and up to 75 percent of patients experience some form of acute pain after surgery. Pain at the incision site usually causes the most trouble. University of Arizona researchers found that resveratrol injections effectively prevented acute postsurgical pain, as well as the development of chronic pain at the incision site.[50]

Thunder God Vine: Rheumatoid Arthritis

Tripterygium wilfordii, known in traditional Chinese medicine as "thunder god vine," appears to be an effective pain reliever, particularly for rheumatoid arthritis. In 2009, researchers at the National Institutes of Health, the University of Texas, and nine rheumatology clinics around the country randomly assigned rheumatoid arthritis patients to either 60 mg of thunder god vine root extract three times per day for six months, or 1 gram of a prescription rheumatoid arthritis medication two times a day for six months. Participants in the study had six or more painful and swollen joints. All were also allowed to take prednisone and nonsteroidal anti-inflammatory drugs (NSAIDs). Patients in both groups experienced side effects, with stomach complaints and digestive symptoms being the most common. About half of participants dropped out of the study before it was completed. However, more dropped out of the prescription drug group than out of the thunder god vine group. Of those who continued treatment for the full six months, 65 percent of the thunder god vine group saw improvements in joint pain, joint function, and inflammation, while just 36 percent of those who took the prescription drug experienced improvements.[51]

Turmeric: Inflammation and Pain

Curcuma longa, better known as turmeric, is the spice that gives curry its bright yellow color and distinctive earthy, slightly bitter, slightly hot peppery flavor and mustardy smell. It is one of the three common components of traditional curry spice (together with coriander and cumin, and sometimes red chili pepper). It is also an important and time-honored ayurvedic remedy for pain. Turmeric is a perfect example of a natural and effective COX-2 inhibitor, and you can take up to 200 mg of it a day to help relieve inflammation and pain. One of its consitutents, curcumin, appears to work especially well for rheumatoid arthritis patients; in a recent study, patients who took curcumin significantly improved their pain.[52] In fact, there are so many studies on turmeric for inflammatory conditions that it seems we could devote the rest of the book to it.

Valerian: Insomnia

Valeriana officinalis is a popular European medicine used for its mild sedative and tranquilizing properties and for help with insomnia. The herb's central nervous system activity is largely ascribed to the constituents of its volatile oils. It is a popular sleep remedy; 2 to 3 grams of the dried root one or more times a day helps combat restlessness and nervous disturbance of sleep.

One study of 128 subjects with varying sleep difficulties compared the effects of an herbal preparation containing *Valeriana officinalis* as one of a mixture of herbs, a valerian-only extract (400 mg), and a placebo. Both valerian preparations produced a significant decrease in insomnia scores and improved sleep quality.[53] In another study, subjects with sleep difficulties received two pills they took on consecutive nights. Both pills contained hops and lemon balm, but one pill contained only 4 mg of valerian and the other contained a full 400 mg dose. Seventy-eight percent of the subjects preferred full-dose valerian, 15 percent preferred the low-dose valerian, and 7 percent had no preference.[54]

BOUNDARY TYPES:
WHO BENEFITS AND WHY

As you know by now, boundary types are how we define and distinguish what is *in here* versus what is *out there*. When it comes to vitamins, nutritional foods, and herbs (or dietary supplements), you are literally taking something from out there and ingesting it in here. You are using digestive and metabolic processes in your body designed for processing any substance that you take in from the environment—including foods, supplementary nutrients, and medicines. While boundary type does not appear to be a primary factor influencing therapeutic effects of vitamins and nutritional foods, your mental state (reflective of your boundary type) may influence the processes of digestion, as well determining your susceptibility to certain gastrointestinal disorders such as IBS (making an understanding of nutritional health even more pertinent). But in the end, everybody (and *every body*) has to eat, and eating well includes an understanding of the benefits of vitamins, herbal remedies, and nutritional foods for everyone.

Some have studied the vibrational and healing energies of plants, and remedies derived therefrom, which could be connected to your health based on how those energies interact with the tendencies of your boundary type. Contemporary research has studied herbal remedies basically as if they were drugs, in the same kinds of clinical trial studies that are considered to provide the "best" possible evidence. The good news is that clinical trial evidence shows dozens of herbs are safe and effective for pain and inflammation and the kinds of conditions we discuss in this book. The bad news is that modern medicine and research does not factor in the mind-body component of nutrition, studying and working with only the physical aspects. So we do not yet have scientific evidence of which boundary types work better with certain dietary supplements and nutritional foods. However, because appropriate use of vitamins, nutritional foods, and herbal remedies is essential for everybody, being mindful of this can help keep our bodies healthy and more amenable to the treatments and practices previously outlined for your boundary type.

12

Essential Oils and Aromatherapy

Aromatherapy is a method of treating bodily ailments using essential plant oils. *Aroma* arises from an aromatic compound, defined in chemical terms as belonging to the closed-chain class of organic compounds or benzene derivatives; *therapy* is defined as a treatment used to combat a disease or abnormal condition. Essential oils are oils that form the odiferous part of plants; they are ethereal, suggesting not only a chemical constituent but also a celestial, spirit-like, or airy quality. On the basis of these definitions, *aromatherapy* is a treatment using a range of organic compounds in which odor or fragrance plays an important part. Jean Valnet (1920–1995), a French surgeon who did pioneering work in this field, spoke of the medicinal uses of essential oils, which he used as antiseptics in the treatment of wounded soldiers during World War II,[1] while Robert Tisserand, a contemporary English aromatherapist, compares the essential oils in plants to the blood in an animal.[2]

Forgotten and ignored for many years, the art and science of using aromatic essences are finally now coming into their own. Many people are no longer willing to be treated except by natural therapies, and this includes plants and their essences. It is evident that both the scientific and the more subtle qualities of aromatherapy are important to those working with plant essential oils.

Aromatherapy appears to be one of the fastest-growing complementary therapies in the United Kingdom. This growth includes not only training in and practice of aromatherapy but also the production of essential oils. In the United Kingdom it is difficult to pick up a magazine or watch a program on alternative medicine that does not mention aromatherapy.

Aromatherapy gradually is becoming more accepted in the orthodox medical field as a treatment to enhance both physical and psychological aspects of patient care. Aromatherapy, as part of therapeutic massage, usually the Swedish style, is now taught to massage therapists and physiotherapists as part of their professional training. Over a hundred English-language books have been published on the topic of aromatherapy in the last twenty years, indicating increasing interest in this subject. Unfortunately, many of these books do not add much new research-based scientific information about essential oils. Some notable exceptions are Pierre Franchomme and Daniel Pénoël, who give detailed chemical analysis of each oil and the indications and contraindications for each in their book *L'aromathérapie exactement;* Robert Tisserand, in his book *The Art of Aromatherapy;* and Tisserand and Rodney Young in their book *Essential Oil Safety,* which includes the available research on essential oils, their chemical constituents, and the clinical practice of aromatherapy. In addition, there is, fortunately, an increasing amount of scientific research being done worldwide as a result of the growing interest in the health benefits of plant essences.

A FRAGRANT HISTORY

The use of aromatic substances and essential oils for health, spiritual, cosmetic, and ceremonial purposes is a long-established tradition that goes back to the ancient Chinese, Indian, Egyptian, Greek, and Roman civilizations. In Egypt, Nefertum was the god of perfumes, incense, and fragrant oils. He was the son of Ptah, a creator god, and Sekmet, the goddess of fiery protection, healing, and alchemical distillation. A hymn to Nefertum describes him as the "Lord of oils and ungents, the soul of life," who smells the soul of the lotus and purifies the body. In

Egyptian life, fragrance was a means of communication between the gods and humanity, offering health to the living and assisting the dead in the next life.[3] There was some overlap between the use of aromatic products for spiritual well-being, health, and beauty. King Ramses III reportedly burned two million blocks of incense during the thirty years of his reign.[4] The medicinal properties of aromatic oils were well understood during later Egyptian periods, and the wide range of essential oils in use then included frankincense, myrrh, cedarwood, henna, and juniper. For example, the essence of cedarwood was prepared by heating it in clay vessels covered by a layer of woolen fibers. These fibers were then squeezed, allowing the essence to be extracted.[5] When the tomb of Tutenkhamun was discovered in 1922, vases were discovered in the tomb that upon analysis were found to contain ointments of frankincense in a base of animal fat. The scent was apparently faint but still in evidence.[6]

The ancient Hebrews probably gained knowledge of aromatic oils from having been the slaves of the Egyptians. Biblical evidence of the use of aromatic substances is present in both the Hebrew Bible and the New Testament: God commanded Moses to make a holy anointing oil of myrrh, cinnamon, calamus, cassia, and olive oil (Exodus 30:22–25); frankincense and myrrh were brought to the baby Jesus by the Three Magi (Matthew 2:11).

The ancient Greeks used aromatic essences both for medicine and for perfumes. Hippocrates expounded the virtues of a daily bath and a scented massage to maintain health and well-being. Aristotle argued that pleasant smells contribute to the well-being of humanity. The Roman poet Lucretius described the particles of pleasant smells as being smooth and round, whereas particles of unpleasant smells were barbed and prickly.

Popular opinion claims that the Arabs discovered how to distill oils from plants during the Middle Ages, with the tenth-century Persian polymath Avicenna given credit for this achievement.[7] However, an Italian research party led by Dr. Paolo Povesti, the director of the International Biocosmetic Research Center in Milan, found a perfectly preserved terra-cotta distillation apparatus or still in the Taxila Museum in the Punjab in Pakistan, at the foot of the Himalayas. It was used for beauty products and dated back five thousand years, to the Indus Valley civilization.[8]

The Middle Ages saw a rise in the use of plant oils both as perfume and as medicine. Catherine de Medici, wife of King Henry II, made the use of aromatic substances for ailments and perfumery fashionable. Her perfumer, Cosimo Ruggieri, not only assisted her with her health and beauty needs but was also able to prepare much less pleasant substances to help dispose of her enemies. During this time aromatic oils were also used to block out the smell of poor hygiene and ward off infection from various pestilences; the pomander, a ball made of perfume that was worn or carried in a globular case that was hung from a neck chain or belt or attached to the girdle, as well as the fragrant tops placed on walking sticks, were commonly used for this purpose. In 1589, a German pharmacopoeia listed eighty essential oils for treating different conditions, and lavender essence was first prepared in France at this time.[9]

Native American shamans were, and are, no strangers to the use of herbs and aromatics. The *perfumeros,* or healers, bathed their patients in scents and by the skillful use of aromatic substances could transform the auric field, the energetic or emotional envelope that surrounds a person. The blowing of tobacco smoke over a person, combined with a perfume, also was seen as having curative powers. The use of fragrance enabled transformations in religious, magical, and healing rituals. An ancient connection exists between fumigating and perfuming in these cultures.[10]

The first recorded use of the term *aromathérapie* was by the French chemist and scholar René-Maurice Gattefossé, in his 1937 book *Aromathérapie: Les Huiles Essentielles, Hormones Végétales.* Gattefossé, considered by many to be the father of the modern-day scientific use of essential oils, first became interested in the study of essential oils after an accident in his laboratory. In 1910, Gattefossé burnt his hand badly after a chemical explosion. He immediately applied some lavender essential oil that was close by. The burn healed with remarkable speed and without infection or scarring. Amazed at this result, Gattefossé began to investigate the properties of essential oils. He was the first person to analyze and record the individual chemical components in each oil, classifying the oils according to their properties (e.g., analgesic, antitoxic, antiseptic, tonifying, stimulating, calming).[11]

Gattefossé subsequently carried out experiments in military hospitals during World War I. He claimed to achieve remarkable results using essential oils, preventing gangrene, curing burns, and obtaining cicatrization far more quickly than usual. However, after the war his methods came under professional scrutiny and were largely abandoned.[12]

Madame Marguerite Maury (1895–1968) was among the first to study and use the effects of essential oils absorbed through the skin. An Austrian-born biochemist, nurse, and surgical assistant, Maury became interested in the use of essential oils after reading a book written in 1838 by a Dr. Chabenes titled *Les grandes possibilités par les matières odoriferantes* (The Great Possibilities of Aromatic Substances); the author was the man who later become the teacher of Gattefossé. Maury promoted the modern-day use of massage with essential oils, the aromatherapy massage, and began teaching aromatherapy, opening the first aromatherapy clinics in France and Switzerland. In 1961 she published *Le capital jeunessee* in France, a book that was published in England in 1964 as *The Secret of Life and Youth* (currently in print as *Marguerite Maury's Guide to Aromatherapy: The Secret of Life and Youth*).

Madame Maury's research into the cutaneous application of essential oils began the teaching of aromatherapy in the 1950s as it is still taught today. She identified two uses of aromatherapy in France: (1) as part of allopathy in its use by doctors, and (2) as a beauty treatment in the form of massage. She also acknowledged the more subtle aspects of aromatherapy and mentioned its link to vibratory medicine. She influenced Micheline Arcier, a well-known aromatherapist in London who met Madame Maury at a beauty conference in 1959. Arcier and three other masseuses asked Maury to establish an aromatherapy clinic for them in London in addition to her clinics in Paris and Switzerland. Arcier then began working with the oils and teaching small numbers of masseuses in the 1960s and 1970s. As well, Arcier also met Jean Valnet, who worked and consulted with her, beginning the development of what is now referred to as the Anglo-Saxon approach to aromatherapy.

During the twentieth century the perfume industry developed separately from the therapeutic field of aromatherapy, with the introduction of such names as Coco Chanel, who launched the famous Chanel No. 5 in 1921. It was she who said that the most mysterious, most human thing is smell. With the subsequent commercial development of the cosmetics industry, the gap between the cosmetic and the therapeutic use of essential oils became increasingly evident. Chanel and her scientific advisers successfully used synthetic products to make modern perfumes. This process separated cosmetics completely from the therapeutic use of essential oils, except perhaps for the good feelings experienced by people wearing and experiencing perfume.

HOW IS IT DONE?

Essential oils are fragrant substances able to impact the body-mind via the olfactory sense, with its direct connections to the brain, including the limbic system and higher brain connections. These connections influence emotions, memory, desire, basic drives, and hormonal responses. The olfactory neurons travel directly to the frontal portions of the brain. For these reasons, inhalation of essential oil fragrance is considered a key aspect of an aromatherapy treatment.

Essential oils are able to impact you on a very subtle vibrational level. Many therapists refer to essential oils as the "life force" of the plant. Thus practices that include different forms of energy medicine such as traditional Chinese and ayurvedic medicines may use essential oils as part of their healing practices.[13]

Essential oils are volatile, fragrant, organic constituents that are obtained from plants either by distillation, which is the most common method, or by cold-pressing, which is used for the extraction of citrus oils only. Oils may be extracted from leaves (eucalyptus, peppermint), flowers (lavender, rose), blossoms (orange blossom or neroli), fruits (lemon, mandarin), grasses (lemongrass), wood (camphor, sandalwood), barks (cinnamon), gum (frankincense), bulbs (garlic, onion), roots (calamus), or dried flower buds (clove). Varying amounts of essential oil can be extracted from a particular plant; for example, 220 pounds of rose petals will yield less than two ounces of essential oil, whereas other plants, such as lavender, lemon, or eucalyptus, give a much greater proportion. This accounts for the variation in price among essential oils. Essential oils come from sources worldwide.

Essential oils might be applied to the body via massage with a vegetable oil, inhaled, used as a compress, mixed into an ointment, or inserted internally through the rectum, vagina, or mouth. The latter method is used chiefly by the medical profession in France.

Essential oils are commonly a mixture of more than a hundred organic compounds that may include esters, alcohols, aldehydes, terpenes, ketones, coumarins, lactones, phenols, oxides, acids, and ethers. Within the oils there might be more of some active constituents than others, which gives the oil its particular therapeutic value. For example, oils containing large amounts of esters (50 to 70 percent), such as neroli (*Citrus aurantium* subsp. *amara* or *bigaradia*), are thought to be calming, whereas other oils, such as that of the tea tree (*Melaleuca alternifolia*), are regarded as antibacterial, antiviral, and immune-system boosters because of the large amounts of alcohol (45 to 50 percent) in their composition.

The technique of liquid gas chromatography is used to identify the quantity of each chemical constituent within the oil.[14] As with grapes grown for wine, the quality of the yield varies according to the climate and other growing conditions of the plant. Lavender oil is popularly thought to be harmless, but according to its chemical type, or chemotype, it might not be suitable for use as a therapeutic oil. *Lavandula angustifolia,* natively grown at approximately 1,000 meters in the French Alps, has a high degree of purity and therapeutic constituents, whereas Spanish lavender, *Lavandula stoechas,* natively grown at sea level by the Mediterranean, contains high quantities of ketones and therefore may be neurotoxic and is contraindicated in pregnant women, babies, and children.[15]

Unless oils are labeled with the full botanical data in Latin, it is impossible to tell whether they are dangerous or contraindicated. Lack of legislation over labeling and quality control of essential oils has contributed to the unease in some health care settings about their use. That essential oils can be purchased at retail stores also gives the general public a false idea as to the relative safety of these oils.

HOW DOES IT WORK?

There are a few underlying principles for treatment with aromatherapy. Many aromatherapists discuss the concept of synergy, that the whole, natural essence is more active than its principal constituents. Those constituents that form a smaller percentage of the whole are often found to be more active than the principal constituent.[16]

The basis of the action of aromatherapy is thought to be the same as that of modern pharmacology, only using smaller doses. The chemical constituents are absorbed into the body, affecting particular physiological processes. Aromatherapy oils are taken into the body through the oral, dermal (skin), rectal, or vaginal routes, or simply by olfaction (smell).

The cutaneous administration of essential oils mixed in a vegetable carrier oil in the form of an aromatherapy massage is a common method of administration in the current approach to aromatherapy. Benefits can be gained not only from the absorption of oils through the skin but also from inhalation of the vapor combined with the physical therapy in the form of massage. Once the oil reaches the upper dermis layer of the skin, it enters the capillary circulation, where the oil can be transported throughout the body.[17] A massage oil made with lavender, for example, penetrates the skin after ten minutes.[18] Blood samples taken at intervals after massage, when analyzed by gas chromatography, showed that two major constituents of lavender oil, linalool and linalyl acetate, reached maximal concentrations twenty minutes after the massage, although traces had been evident at five minutes. Levels returned to baseline after ninety minutes, indicating elimination of lavender from the bloodstream.[19] Other studies support the passage of aromatic compounds through the skin of humans.[20]

A significantly smaller dose is administered to the body through the skin than when given orally.[21] The oral administration of essential oils comes from the current French medical approach to aromatherapy and carries more potential risks of poisoning or irritation to the gastric mucosa if administered by unqualified persons. It might be useful for qualified medical practitioners to get larger doses of essential oils into the body for the treatment of serious infections, but a more detailed knowledge of essential oil toxicology is required for administration via this route than is possessed by the average aromatherapist. It is noteworthy that interest in this form of administration is growing, and there are good opportunities for training in this style of administration in the English language, particularly in Provence, France, with professional trainers such as aromatherapist, author, and educator Rhiannon Lewis and consultant and educator Bob Harris.

Rectal administration of oils in the form of suppositories may be useful for local problems and to avoid the liver-portal system of the body, thus allowing higher systemic concentrations of the oils to be absorbed. Vaginal administration in the form of pessaries or douches also is used for local problems. Simple inhalation of oil is a method used for respiratory conditions, insomnia, and mood elevation and enhancement, or to simply make an environment more pleasant. Steam inhalers can be used for respiratory infections, and a variety of electrical and fan-assisted apparatuses may be used to scent a room. It is not surprising that essential oils are absorbed through inhalation. In fact, it's been proven: inhalation of rosemary oil is associated with a rise in serum levels of 1,8-cineole, a major constituent of rosemary, aromatic compounds of sandalwood, rose, neroli, and lavender all have been shown to be present in the blood after inhalation.[22] Overexposure to oils absorbed by this method can result in headaches, fatigue, or allergic reactions such as streaming eyes and skin problems.

The additional influence of touch in the form of massage is a major aspect of aromatherapy treatment when the oils are administered via the skin. One study was able to show additional psychological benefit, including reduction in anxiety, for patients who had aromatherapy massage with essential oil of neroli compared with those who had massage with a plain vegetable oil.[23] Other studies have shown positive psychological benefits from massage, including positive subjective response,[24] the perceived state of relaxation,[25] reported pleasurable feelings,[26] and an improvement in the perceived level of anxiety.[27] The importance of massage for both relaxation and the release of physical and psychological stress should not be underestimated and can be seen only as a positive aid to the administration of essential oils when administered appropriately.

It is suggested that aromatherapy would not have gained its rapid increase in popularity if the oils were not fragrant, thus affecting mood and emotions. Several references have already been made to the inextricable link between the development of human biology, the sense of smell, and the importance of aromas. Sigmund Freud developed the idea of "organic repression" of the sense of smell. He attributed this to the upright gait, which elevates the nose from the ground, where it had enjoyed pleasurable sensations previously.[28] This repression may not be complete, but many people have a diminished sense of smell, a sense more vital to the survival of animals than humans. It may be this need to satisfy pleasurable sensations via the sense of smell that is attracting so many people to aromatherapy today.

The human response to aromas is associated with olfaction, naturally. The neurons of the olfactory system, which are the chemical senses of the body, rest in that part of the midbrain known as the limbic system. The structures of the brain's limbic system extend from the midbrain through the hypothalamus into the basal forebrain, which is concerned not only with visceral functions but also with emotional expression. The cortical and medial nuclei of the amygdala, a body situated within this system, receive information from the olfactory system. The basolateral nuclei are involved with the expression of emotion,[29] and therefore aromatherapy's effect on emotion and psychological state is not surprising.[30]

Medical Aromatherapy

In addition to their more cosmetic abilities to enhance self-image and self-esteem, essential oils have a variety uses in a medical setting: burn healing, relief of insomnia and restlessness, infection and general wound healing, pain and discomfort relief, relaxation, stress and anxiety relief, immune-function stimulation, and treatment for constipation.

When essential oils are integrated into medical environments alongside mainstream care to address particular patient challenges, the practice is often termed *clinical aromatherapy*. It effectively represents a merging of both holistic and medical styles that are adapted to individual needs. While most interventions in medical environments still tend toward the use of the lower-dose external and inhalation methods, as in holistic aromatherapy, there is an increasing trend toward and acceptance of using more intensive interventions when necessary for particular clinical challenges, such as pain management, odor control, wound care, oral care, and treatment of infection. This style of aromatherapy is characterized by the following:

- Clinical aromatherapy's role as a holistic approach, especially with regard to well-being and anxiety reduction, is a main focus.
- Essential oils are prescribed to treat a range of predominantly physical disorders (e.g., infection, contagions, pain, and inflammation).
- Administration methods include topical, oral, sublingual, rectal, vaginal, and inhalational. Most interventions involve topical (including inside the mouth) application or inhalation. Ingestion or rectal administration is less frequent.
- Dosages vary widely according to requirements but are generally higher or more intensive than those employed in holistic aromatherapy.
- Essential oils and other active agents such as herbal tinctures might be used in combination, and they are usually administered by the patient him- or herself, but under the guidance of the practitioner.
- Interventions are often brief and specifically focused (e.g., anxiety management, relief of nausea, oral care, wound care, pain relief).
- Clinical aromatherapy is usually delivered by a trained practitioner as part of regular health care procedures.

CHEMICAL COMPONENTS OF ESSENTIAL OILS AND THEIR THERAPEUTIC ACTIONS*

Chemical Component	Therapeutic Action
aldehydes	anti-infectious, litholytic, calming
ketones	mucolytic, litholytic, cicatris healing, calming
esters	antispasmodic, calming
sesquiterpenes	antihistaminic, antiallergic
coumarins, lactones	balancing, calming
C15 and C20	estrogen-like action
aromatic acids	anti-infectious
aldehydes	immunostimulant
phenols	anti-infectious
alcohols	immunostimulant
oxides	expectorant, antiparasitic
phenyl methyl ethers	anti-infectious, antispasmodic
terpenes	antiseptic, cortisone-like action

*Adapted from Franchomme and Pénoîl, L'aromathérapie exactement.

THE PROVEN EFFECTIVENESS OF AROMATHERAPY

Analgesic properties are attributed to some essential oils. One study demonstrated that lemongrass leaves produced a dose-dependent analgesia. Both dermal and oral doses of one of its constituents, myrcene, were administered with similar effect. Myrcene, a constituent of other oils, including rosemary, lavender, juniper, and ylang-ylang, was credited with this effect.[31]

In the United Kingdom, the evaluation of aromatherapy for pain and neurological disorders has included three recent scientific Cochrane reviews: (1) pain relief in cases of cancer and palliative care;[32] (2) the effectiveness of aromatherapy for dementia;[33] and (3) complementary and alternative therapies for pain management in labor that include aromatherapy.[34] A 2001 survey of aromatherapists ascertained their treatment of patients with rheumatic disease symptoms and found that they frequently prescribe both English and German chamomile (*Chamaemelum nobile* and *Matricaria chamomilla,* respectively) to help with pain and inflamed joints.

Cancer and Palliative Care

In the United Kingdom, aromatherapy and massage are the most popular complementary therapies for people with cancer. A 2012 survey assessed access to CAM therapies for people with cancer within the British National Health Service. A total of 142 units were identified across England, Wales, Scotland, and Northern Ireland, which provided sixty-two different CAM therapies. Counseling was the most widely provided therapy (available at 82.4 percent of identified units), followed by reflexology (62.0 percent), aromatherapy (59.1 percent), Reiki (43.0 percent), and massage (42.2 percent).[35]

Stress Reduction and Relaxation

A 1991 study involved perhaps the most extensive research on essential oils using animal models. After one hour of inhaling an essential oil or fragrance compound, mice became sedated by sandalwood, rose, neroli, and lavender.[36] Another 1988 study involving human subjects examined the psychological, autonomic, endocrine, and immune consequences of a relaxant odor (lavender), a stimulant odor (lemon), and a no-odor control (water). It was found that inhalation of the essential oils led to a change in brain-wave activity, which generally supports the claims of stimulation and relaxation made about specific essential oils.[37]

Some essential oils with sedative properties, such as frankincense (*Boswellia carterii*), may help with sedation in the dying and reduce the need for morphine. Ancient practices involving anointing the dying with frankincense may have been as much to help the dying person as to prevent the spread of microbes.

In the United Kingdom, studies on the effects of essential oils have been performed in intensive-care units and palliative-care and senior settings. Some of these trials found psychological benefits from aromatherapy, in addition to massage. In a four-day study of a hundred patients in intensive care, foot massage with neroli oil was more effective in reducing anxiety than massage with a plain vegetable oil.[38] A 1993 study in which patients were massaged with two different lavender essential oils, *Lavandula angustifolia* (true lavender) and *Lavandula latifolia* (spike lavender), found a difference in the effects of the two oils.[39] Spike lavender had a more significant effect than true lavender. True lavender grows naturally at high altitudes, while spike lavender thrives more at lower altitudes. The altitude difference in growing environments explains why spike lavender oil contains more camphor, the chemical responsible for its sweet herbaceous smell, while true lavender oil has very little to no camphor. Due to its stronger camphor content, spike lavender oil is said to provide more potent analgesia and typically is excellent for relief of sore throats or coughing. Topically, it may work as an insect repellent and as a salve to help ease pains and other discomfort caused by arthritis. In an unpublished 1992 study, an investigation of 122 patients in intensive care measured the effects of massage with lavender oil compared with a plain oil massage. The physiological changes were not significant, but positive psychological changes resulted for those massaged with essential oil more so than for those who received the plain oil massage.[40]

In a study of over fifty patients in a center for palliative care, the effects of three aromatherapy massages given weekly with or without the essential oil of Roman chamomile, *Chamaemelum nobile*, were examined. Anxiety for all patients improved.[41] In a small study of four patients on a long-stay elder-care ward, researchers assessed sleep over three consecutive two-week periods—the first period with night sedation, the second without, and the third with lavender diffused into the air at set intervals. Sleep was poorer in the second week, and in the third week sleep was as good as in the first week.[42]

Wound Healing

As recent as 2016 many studies show the incredible wound-healing and anti-inflammatory effects of essential oils and aromatic extracts, including lavender (*Lavandula angustifolia*), mugwort (*Artemisia vulgaris*), sage (*Salvia officinalis*), and everlasting flower (*Helichrysum italicum* ssp. *serotinum*).

Anecdotal reports from mothers indicate that lavender oil helps relieve perineal discomfort after childbirth. Following this, a randomized trial involving 635 postpartum women had each woman adding six drops of either pure lavender oil, a synthetic lavender oil that smelled like the other, or an inert compound to a bath daily. Perineal pain was slightly reduced in the pure lavender group.

BOUNDARY TYPES: WHO BENEFITS AND WHY

Plant essential oils and their use in aromatherapy are remarkable for crossing the boundaries of your body. They are rubbed on the skin (sometimes via massage and bodywork), placed on the body at key points, or simply inhaled through the nostrils into the lungs. As plant constituents, their effects on the physical body have been studied in much the same way as have herbal remedies showing remarkable benefits for pain, inflammation, and other conditions described in this book.

But there is another dimension to this therapy for the mind-body where boundary types may come into play. When typically used as part of bodywork and massage, plant essential oil therapy may bring up sensitivities with thin boundary types—who are typically more sensitive to the environment. The use of plant essential oils for thin boundary types may create actual physical discomfort such as skin or nasal irritation and/or emotional sensitivities—especially due to the powerful connections of smell and aromas with the brain and memory.

Thick boundary people, who like to keep things out there, may not be as comfortable with touching and being anointed with oils on the naked skin. They (especially men) may also be resistant to being perfumed or using scents. Again, it is a question of your therapist working with your comfort levels—and you providing ongoing feedback to the therapist—to find the right type of usage and the right scents to make oils work for your individual constitution.

Your sense of smell is the most potent (and primitive) power of your body. Smell allows us to detect what is *out there,* often better than any other sense (as is the case with most terrestrial animals). Sense of smell is also directly wired into what is *in there.* In that sense, there may be no boundaries for the powerful technique of aromatherapy. If it smells right, do it.

HOW TO FIND A PRACTITIONER

In the United States there are now two organizations representing standards in training in aromatherapy: the National Association for Holistic Aromatherapy (NAHA), which has over four thousand members, and the Aromatherapy Registration Council, which has set a national exam for registration. Some colleges and universities offer postgraduate courses in aromatherapy for nurses. Each state develops its own legislation in relation to practice. As with any other kind of service provider, the best way to find a good aromatherapist is through referrals from your health care providers, family, colleagues, and friends. When choosing a practitioner, it is important to consider his or her education and training, experience, and philosophy of care. You can find a qualified aromatherapist by state on the NAHA website (www.naha.org) or at the Aromatherapy Registration Council website (www.aromatherapycouncil.org).

In Europe and the United Kingdom, the health benefits of aromatherapy have been widely embraced for many years, as is reflected in the many settings in which it is found: intensive-care units, palliative-care settings, coronary-care units, hospices, renal units, pediatric units, neurologic units, midwifery units, HIV/AIDS units, learning-disability settings, geriatric units, cancer units, burn units, rheumatology units, and wound clinics. Aromatherapists who work in practices with general medical practitioners generally do so on a session-by-session basis, with the physician maintaining clinical responsibility for the patient referred to the aromatherapist. In these kinds of orthodox health care settings, services are provided by lay aromatherapists and increasingly by nurses or physiotherapists with aromatherapy training.

The Boundary Questionnaire

Below is the full-length Boundary Questionnaire developed by Dr. Ernest Hartmann. Afterward is a key for you to score your responses.

Note: While the statements are phrased in a general way, none of them is meant as a value judgment. There are no right or wrong responses. Consider these statements merely as prompts intended to sound you out on where you are right now in your life.

That being said, please rate each of the following statements from 0 to 4. A rating of 0 indicates "not at all" or "not at all true of me," whereas a rating of 4 indicates "yes, definitely" or "very true of me." Try to respond to all of the statements as quickly as you can.

1. When I wake up in the morning, I am not sure whether I am really awake for a few minutes.   0 1 2 3 4

2. I have had unusual reactions to alcohol.   0 1 2 3 4

3. My feelings blend into one another.   0 1 2 3 4

4. I am very close to my childhood feelings.   0 1 2 3 4

5. I am very careful about what I say to people until I get to know them really well.   0 1 2 3 4

6. I am very sensitive to other people's feelings.   0 1 2 3 4

7. I like to pigeonhole things as much as possible.   0 1 2 3 4

8. I like solid music with a definite beat. 0 1 2 3 4

9. I think children have a special sense of joy and wonder that is later often lost. 0 1 2 3 4

10. In an organization, everyone should have a definite place and a specific role. 0 1 2 3 4

11. People of different nations are basically very much alike. 0 1 2 3 4

12. There are a great many forces influencing us that science does not understand at all. 0 1 2 3 4

13. I have dreams, daydreams, or nightmares in which my body or someone else's body is being stabbed, injured, or torn apart. 0 1 2 3 4

14. I have had unusual reactions to marijuana. 0 1 2 3 4

15. Sometimes I don't know whether I am thinking or feeling. 0 1 2 3 4

16. I can remember things from when I was less than three years old. 0 1 2 3 4

17. I expect other people to keep a certain distance. 0 1 2 3 4

18. I think I would be a good psychotherapist. 0 1 2 3 4

19. I keep my desk and worktable neat and well organized. 0 1 2 3 4

20. I think it might be fun to wear medieval armor. 0 1 2 3 4

21. A good teacher needs to help a child remain special. 0 1 2 3 4

22. When making a decision, you shouldn't let your feelings get in the way. 0 1 2 3 4

23. Being dressed neatly and cleanly is very important. 0 1 2 3 4

24. There is time for thinking and there is a time for feeling; they should be kept separate. 0 1 2 3 4

25. My daydreams don't always stay in control. 0 1 2 3 4

26. I have had unusual reactions to coffee or tea. 0 1 2 3 4

27. For me, things are black or white; there are no shades of gray. 0 1 2 3 4

28. I had a difficult and complicated childhood.   0 1 2 3 4

29. When I get involved with someone, I know exactly who I am and who the other person is. We may cooperate, but we maintain our separate selves.   0 1 2 3 4

30. I am easily hurt.   0 1 2 3 4

31. I get to appointments right on time.   0 1 2 3 4

32. I like heavy, solid clothing.   0 1 2 3 4

33. Children and adults have a lot in common. They should give themselves a chance to be together without any strict roles.   0 1 2 3 4

34. In getting along with other people in an organization, it is very important to be flexible and adaptable.   0 1 2 3 4

35. I believe many of the world's problems could be solved if only people trusted each other more.   0 1 2 3 4

36. Either you are telling the truth or you are lying; that's all there is to it.   0 1 2 3 4

37. I spend a lot of time daydreaming, fantasizing, or in reverie.   0 1 2 3 4

38. I am afraid I may fall apart completely.   0 1 2 3 4

39. I like to have beautiful experiences without analyzing them or trying to understand them in detail.   0 1 2 3 4

40. I have definite plans for my future. I can lay out pretty well what I expect year by year at least for the next few years.   0 1 2 3 4

41. I can usually tell what another person is thinking or feeling without anyone saying anything.   0 1 2 3 4

42. I am unusually sensitive to loud noises and to bright lights.   0 1 2 3 4

43. I am good at keeping accounts and keeping track of my money.   0 1 2 3 4

44. I like stories that have a definite beginning, middle, and end.   0 1 2 3 4

45. I think an artist must in part remain a child.   0 1 2 3 4

46. A good organization is one in which all the lines of responsibility are precise and clearly established.   0 1 2 3 4

47. Each nation should be clear about its interests and its boundaries, as well as the interests and boundaries of other nations.   0 1 2 3 4

48. There is a place for everything, and everything should be in its place.   0 1 2 3 4

49. Every time something frightening happens to me, I have nightmares, fantasies, or flashbacks involving the frightening event.   0 1 2 3 4

50. I feel unsure of who I am at times.   0 1 2 3 4

51. At times I feel happy and sad all at once.   0 1 2 3 4

52. I have a clear memory of my past. I could tell you pretty well what happened year by year.   0 1 2 3 4

53. When I get involved with someone, we sometimes get too close.   0 1 2 3 4

54. I am a very sensitive person.   0 1 2 3 4

55. I like things to be spelled out precisely and specifically.   0 1 2 3 4

56. I think a good teacher must remain in part a child.   0 1 2 3 4

57. I like paintings and drawings with clear outlines and no blurred edges.   0 1 2 3 4

58. A good relationship is one in which everything is clearly defined and spelled out.   0 1 2 3 4

59. People are totally different from each other.   0 1 2 3 4

60. When I wake up, I wake up quickly and am absolutely sure I am awake.   0 1 2 3 4

61. At times I have felt as if I were coming apart.   0 1 2 3 4

62. My thoughts blend into one another.   0 1 2 3 4

63. I had a difficult and complicated adolescence.   0 1 2 3 4

64. Sometimes it's scary when one gets too involved with another person.   0 1 2 3 4

65. I enjoy soaking up atmosphere even if I don't understand exactly what's going on.   0 1 2 3 4

67.* I like paintings or drawings with soft and blurred edges.   0 1 2 3 4

68. A good parent has to be a bit of a child too.   0 1 2 3 4

69. I cannot imagine marrying or living with someone of another religion.   0 1 2 3 4

70. It is very hard truly to empathize with another person because people are so different.   0 1 2 3 4

71. All important thought involves feelings too.   0 1 2 3 4

72. I have dreams, daydreams, or nightmares in which I see isolated body parts—arms, legs, heads, and so on.   0 1 2 3 4

73. Things around me seem to change their size and shape.   0 1 2 3 4

74. I can easily imagine myself to be an animal or what it might be like to be an animal.   0 1 2 3 4

75. I feel very separate and distinct from everyone else.   0 1 2 3 4

76. When I am in a new situation, I try to find out precisely what is going on and what the rules are as soon as possible.   0 1 2 3 4

77. I enjoy(ed) geometry; there are simple, straightforward rules and everything fits.   0 1 2 3 4

78. A good parent must be able to empathize with his or her children, and to be their friend and playmate at the same time.   0 1 2 3 4

79. I cannot imagine living with or marrying a person of another race.   0 1 2 3 4

80. People are so different that I never know what someone else is thinking or feeling.   0 1 2 3 4

81. Beauty is a very subjective thing. I know what I like, but I wouldn't expect anyone else to agree.   0 1 2 3 4

---

*There was no question 66 on Dr. Hartmann's original Boundary Questionnaire, but no worries—it's an old oversight from his early work and he and his colleagues have worked around it. Nothing is actually omitted.

82. In my daydreams, people kind of merge into one another or one person turns into another.   0 1 2 3 4

83. My body sometimes seems to change its size or shape.   0 1 2 3 4

84. I get overinvolved in things.   0 1 2 3 4

85. When something happens to a friend of mine or a lover, it is almost as if it happened to me.   0 1 2 3 4

86. When I work on a project, I don't like to tie myself down to a definite outline. I rather like to let my mind wander.   0 1 2 3 4

87. Good solid frames are very important for a picture or painting.   0 1 2 3 4

88. I think children need strict discipline.   0 1 2 3 4

89. People are happier with their own kind than mixing with others.   0 1 2 3 4

90. "East is east and west is west and never the twain shall meet." (Kipling)   0 1 2 3 4

91. There are definite rules and standards, which one can learn, about what is and is not beautiful.   0 1 2 3 4

92. In my dreams, people sometimes merge into each other or become other people.   0 1 2 3 4

93. I believe I am influenced by forces that no one can understand.   0 1 2 3 4

94. When I read something, I get so involved it can be difficult to get back to reality.   0 1 2 3 4

95. I trust people easily.   0 1 2 3 4

96. When I am working on a project, I make a careful, detailed outline and then follow it closely.   0 1 2 3 4

97. The movies and TV shows I like the best are the ones with good guys and bad guys, and you always know who they are.   0 1 2 3 4

98. If we open ourselves to the world, we find that things go better than expected.   0 1 2 3 4

99. Most people are sane; some people are crazy; there is no in-between.   0 1 2 3 4

100. I have had déjà vu experiences.   0 1 2 3 4

101. I have a very definite sense of space around me.   0 1 2 3 4

102. When I really get involved in a game or in playing at something, it's sometimes hard when the game stops and the rest of the world begins.   0 1 2 3 4

103. I am a very open person.   0 1 2 3 4

104. I think I would enjoy being an engineer.   0 1 2 3 4

105. There are no sharp dividing lines between normal people, people with problems, and people who are considered psychotic or crazy.   0 1 2 3 4

106. When I listen to music, I get so involved it is sometimes difficult to get back to reality.   0 1 2 3 4

107. I am always at least a little bit on my guard.   0 1 2 3 4

108. I am a down-to-earth, no-nonsense kind of person.   0 1 2 3 4

109. I like houses with flexible spaces, where you can shift things around and make different uses out of the same rooms.   0 1 2 3 4

110. Success is largely a matter of good organization and keeping good records.   0 1 2 3 4

111. Everyone is a little crazy at times.   0 1 2 3 4

112. I have daymares.   0 1 2 3 4

113. I awake from one dream into another.   0 1 2 3 4

114. Time slows down and speeds up for me. Time passes very differently on different occasions.   0 1 2 3 4

115. I feel at one with the world.   0 1 2 3 4

116. Sometimes I meet someone and trust him or her so completely that I can share just about everything about myself at the first meeting.   0 1 2 3 4

117. I think I would enjoy being the captain of a ship.   0 1 2 3 4

118. Good fences make good neighbors.   0 1 2 3 4

119. My dreams are so vivid that even later I can't tell them from waking reality.　　　0 1 2 3 4

120. I have often had the experience of different senses coming together. For example, I have felt that I could smell a color, or see a sound, or hear an odor.　　　0 1 2 3 4

121. I read things straight through from beginning to end. (I don't skip or go off on interesting tangents.)　　　0 1 2 3 4

122. I have friends and I have enemies, and I know which are which.　　　0 1 2 3 4

123. I think I would enjoy being some kind of creative artist.　　　0 1 2 3 4

124. A man is a man and a woman is a woman; it is very important to maintain that distinction.　　　0 1 2 3 4

125. I know exactly which parts of town are safe and which parts are unsafe.　　　0 1 2 3 4

126. I have had the experience of not knowing whether I was imagining something or it was actually happening.　　　0 1 2 3 4

127. When I recall a conversation or a piece of music, I hear it just as though it was happening there again right in front of me.　　　0 1 2 3 4

128. I think I would enjoy a really loose, flexible job where I could write my own job description.　　　0 1 2 3 4

129. All men have something feminine in them, and all women have something masculine in them.　　　0 1 2 3 4

130. In my dreams, I have been a person of the opposite sex.　　　0 1 2 3 4

131. I have had the experience of someone calling me or speaking my name, and not being sure whether it was really happening or whether I was imagining it.　　　0 1 2 3 4

132. I can visualize something so vividly that it is just as though it is happening right in front of me.　　　0 1 2 3 4

133. I think I could be a good fortune teller or a medium.　　　0 1 2 3 4

134. In my dreams, I am always myself.　　　0 1 2 3 4

135. I see auras or fields of energy around people.　　　0 1 2 3 4

136. I can easily imagine myself to be someone of the opposite sex. 0 1 2 3 4

137. I like clear, precise borders. 0 1 2 3 4

138. I have had the feeling that someone who is close to me was in danger or was hurt, although I had no ordinary way of knowing it, and later found out that it was true. 0 1 2 3 4

139. I have a very clear and distinct sense of time. 0 1 2 3 4

140. I like houses where rooms have definite walls and each room has a definite function. 0 1 2 3 4

141. I have had dreams that later came true. 0 1 2 3 4

142. I like fuzzy borders. 0 1 2 3 4

143. I have had "out of body" experiences during which my mind seemed to, or actually did, leave my body. 0 1 2 3 4

144. I like straight lines. 0 1 2 3 4

145. I like wavy or curved lines better than I like straight lines. 0 1 2 3 4

146. I feel sure that I can empathize with the very old. 0 1 2 3 4

SCORING THE BOUNDARY QUESTIONNAIRE

A score sheet is presented on pages 236–37. All the statements listed in the left-hand column are "thin" items; the statements in the right-hand column are "thick" items. The differences should be clear from reading the items.

Under each statement number in the left-hand column, enter the response you circled for that item. Under each number in the right-hand column, enter the *inverse* of your response, according to the following table:

$4 = 0$ $3 = 1$ $2 = 2$ $1 = 3$ $0 = 4$

Add the scores entered in both columns to obtain your total for each of the twelve themed categories plus your overall total at the bottom of the score sheet. (On the average, the total for all questions is 250 to 300.)*

It's worth mentioning that one can be a thin or thick boundary person overall and yet have a different type of boundary score within the various categories. No one is reducible to a single location on the boundary spectrum. Each of us is likely to be thin in some respects and thick in others.

BOUNDARY QUESTIONNAIRE SCORE SHEET

	Thin Items Score by adding what you circled from 0–4 for the given question numbers.	Thick Items Score by adding the inverse of what you circled for the given question numbers.	Score
Category 1: Sleeping/waking/dreaming	1, 13, 25, 37, 49, 72, 82, 92, 112, 113, 119, 130	60, 134	_____
Category 2: Unusual experiences	2, 14, 26, 38, 50, 61, 73, 83, 93, 100, 114, 120, 126, 131, 135, 138, 141, 143	(101, though not actually included in the score)	_____
Category 3: Thoughts/feelings/moods	3, 15, 39, 51, 62, 74, 84, 94, 102, 106, 115, 127, 132, 136	27, 139	_____
Category 4: Childhood/adolescence/adulthood	4, 16, 28, 63	40, 52	_____
Category 5: Interpersonal	41, 53, 64, 85, 95, 103, 116, 146	5, 29, 122, 125 (also 17, 75, and 107, though not actually included in the score)	_____
Category 6: Sensitivity	6, 18, 30, 42, 54	no items	_____

*To have your scores automatically calculated, go to www.drmicozzi.com and take the Your Emotional Type survey.

Category 7: Neatness/exactness/ precision	65, 86	7, 19, 31, 43, 55, 76, 96, 108, 121	_____
	Thin Items Score by adding what you circled from 0–4 for the given question numbers.	**Thick Items** Score by adding the inverse of what you circled for the given question numbers.	**Score**
Category 8: Edges/lines/clothing	67, 109, 123, 128, 133, 142, 145	44, 57, 77, 87, 97, 104, 117, 137, 140, 144 (also 8, 20, and 32, though not included in the score)	_____
Category 9: Opinions about children and others	9, 21, 33, 45, 56, 68, 78	88	_____
Category 10: Opinions about organizations and relationships	34, 98	10, 22, 46, 58, 69, 79, 89, 110	_____
Category 11: Opinions about peoples, nations, and groups	11, 35, 105, 111, 129	23, 47, 59, 70, 80, 90, 99, 118, 124	_____
Category 12: Opinions about beauty and truth	12, 71, 81	24, 36, 48, 91	_____

THICK BOUNDARY--------------------**MIDDLE**--------------------------**THIN BOUNDARY**

| 0 | 50 | 100 | 150 | 200 | 250 | 300 | 350 | 400 | 450 | 500 | 550 | 580 |

Notes

INTRODUCTION.
THE PROBLEM OF PAIN

1. University of Wisconsin, "Achieving Balance in State Pain Policy."
2. University of Wisconsin, "Achieving Balance in Federal and State Pain Policy."
3. Ibid.
4. Toblin et al., "Chronic pain."
5. Riddle, Jiranek, and Hayes, "Use."
6. Draucker et al., "Acceptability."
7. Banth and Ardebil, "Effectiveness."
8. Rod, "Observing."
9. Belcaro et al., "Management."
10. Arora et al., "Curcumin."
11. Appelboom, Maes, and Albert, "New curcuma."
12. Merolla et al., "Co-analgesic."
13. Peanpadungrat, "Efficacy."
14. Ibid.; Hill et al., "Fish oil."

1. PAIN AND YOUR EMOTIONAL TYPE

1. Kolata, "Death."
2. Segerdahl et al., "Dorsal."
3. Hartmann, *Dreams,* 228.
4. Ibid., 229.
5. Jawer and Micozzi, *Spiritual.*

2. RELAXATION AND STRESS REDUCTION

1. Selye, *Stress.*
2. Ibid.

3. Jawer and Micozzi, *Spiritual.*

4. Ibid.

5. McCown and Micozzi, *New World.*

6. Ibid.; McCown, Reibel, and Micozzi, *Teaching.*

7. Pearce, *Magical.*

8. Morris, *Human.*

9. Nabi et al., "Increased risk."

10. Jawer and Micozzi, *Your Emotional Type.*

11. Esch et al., "Stress."

12. Johansson et al., "Common."

13. Benson, "Relaxation response."

14. Sacks, "Exercise."

15. Chang et al., "Relaxation."

16. Bhasin et al., "Relaxation."

3. BIOFEEDBACK

1. Häuser et al., "Systematic."

2. Barlow and Durand, *Abnormal.*

3. Harvard Health Publications, "Depression."

4. Mueller et al., "Treatment."

5. Toscano and Cowlings, "Reducing."

4. IMAGERY AND VISUALIZATION

1. Blakeslee, Macknik, and Martinez-Conde, *Sleights.*

2. Kreiman, Koch, and Fried, "Imagery neurons."

3. Ganis, Thompson, and Kosslyn, "Brain areas."

4. Baars and Gage, "Consciousness."

5. Olness and Conroy, "Pilot."

6. Barber, *Hypnosis,* v 282.

7. Green and Green, *Beyond Biofeedback.*

8. Luria, *Mind.*

9. Jordan and Lenington, "Physiological."

10. Barber, Chauncey, and Winer, "Effect"; White, "Salivation."

11. From a personal correspondence with Marc Micozzi.

12. Ibid.

13. Häuser, Hansen, and Enck, "Nocebo phenomena."

14. Ibid.

15. Sloman, "Relaxation."

16. Ghoneim et al., "Tape-recorded."

17. Bennett, "Comparison."

18. Tusek, Church, and Fazio, "Guided."

5. HYPNOSIS

1. Graci and Sexton-Radek, "Treating," 296.
2. Goldsmith, *Franz Anton Mesmer.*
3. Bechtel and Richardson, "Vitalism."
4. Goldsmith, *Franz Anton Mesmer,* 155.
5. Graci and Sexton-Radek, "Treating," 296.
6. Ibid.
7. Ibid.
8. Gosline, "Hypnosis."
9. Spiegel, "Mind prepared."
10. Ibid.
11. Rogovik and Goldman, "Hypnosis."
12. Montgomery, DuHamel, and Redd, "Meta-analysis."
13. Ehrlich, "Hypnotherapy."
14. Ghoneim et al., "Tape-recorded."
15. Enqvist and Fisher, "Preoperative"; Enqvist, Von Konow, and Bystedt, "Stress reduction."
16. Bay and Bay, "Combined therapy."
17. Olness and Gardner, *Hypnosis.*
18. DeBenedittis, Panerai, and Villamira, "Effects."
19. Lindfors et al., "Effects."
20. Lindfors et al., "Long-term."
21. Cyna, McAuliffe, and Andrew, "Hypnosis."
22. Cyna, "Hypno-analgesia."
23. Martin, "Effects."
24. Gordon, "Fresh Face."
25. Perlman, "Dentistry."
26. Montgomery et al., "Effectiveness."
27. Yazici et al., "Effectiveness."

6. MEDITATION AND YOGA

1. Gehl and Micozzi, *Science.*
2. Quoted in foreword of McCown, Reibel, and Micozzi, *Teaching.*
3. McCown and Micozzi, *New World.*
4. Ibid.
5. Kaplan, Goldenberg, and Nadeau, "Impact."
6. Dunn, Hartigan, and Mikulas, "Concentration."
7. Mills and Allen, "Mindfulness."
8. Carlson et al., "Effects."
9. McCown and Micozzi, "Mind-body."
10. Cooper and Aygen, "Effect."

11. Brooks and Scarano, "Transcendental"; Kabat-Zinn et al., "Four-year."
12. Staples, "Yoga."
13. Prentiss, *Embodiment,* 211.
14. Shah, "Jain," 21.
15. Feuerstein, "History."
16. Ricci, "T.K.V."
17. Ibid.
18. Goldberg, *Goddess.*
19. Woodyard, "Exploring."
20. Keniger et al., "What."
21. Jaju et al., "Effects"; Donesky-Cuenco et al., "Yoga"; Danucalov et al., "Cardiorespiratory." Suggested further reading: Chaya and Nagendra, "Long-term."
22. Benson et al., "Continuous." For more on this topic see Kuvalaynanda, "Oxygen."
23. Woodyard, "Exploring."
24. Desikachar, Bragdon, and Bossart, "Yoga."
25. Manjunath and Telles, "Influence."
26. Woodyard, "Exploring."
27. Gothe, Kramer, and McAuley, "Effects."
28. Staples, "Yoga," 332–43.
29. Gura, "Yoga."
30. Bartlett et al., "Yoga."
31. Woodyard, "Exploring."
32. Kotchen, "Historical."
33. Heath, "Waste."
34. Hewett et al., "Examination."

7. SPIRITUAL HEALING

1. Braud, "Human"; Jahn and Dunne, "Precognitive."
2. Herbert, *Quantum,* 249.
3. Solfvin, "Mental."
4. Wilber, "Psychologic."
5. LeShan, *Medium.*
6. Stellar et al., "Positive."
7. Pargamont, Koenig, and Perez, "Many."
8. Koenig, "Religion."
9. Ellis, Vinson, and Ewigman, "Addressing."
10. Byrd, "Positive."
11. Harris et al., "Randomized."
12. Matthews, Marlowe, and MacNutt, "Effects."

13. Abbot et al., "Spiritual."
14. Targ and Levine, "Efficacy."
15. Kinney et al., "Holistic."

8. MASSAGE AND BODYWORK

1. Pemberton, "Physiology."
2. Chaitow, *Muscle.*
3. Lewit and Simons, "Myofascial."
4. Chaitow and DeLany, *Upper;* Chaitow and DeLany, *Lower.*
5. Lowe, "Orthopedic."
6. Ibid.
7. Donoyama, Munakata, and Shibasaki, "Effects"; Donoyama, Satoh, and Hamano, "Effects"; Donoyama et al., "Physical"; Field, "Massage"; Richards, Gibson, and Overton-McCoy, "Effects."
9. Wells, Pasero, and McCaffery, "Improving"; Espi-Lopez et al., "Effect."
10. Brody, "Let."
11. Frye in a personal communication with Micozzi.
12. American Masssage Therapy Association (AMTA), "Industry fact sheet."
13. Ibid.
14. AMTA, "Living right."
15. AMTA, "Use of massage therapy."
16. AMTA, "Living right."

9. CHIROPRACTIC

1. Wilk v. American Medical Association.
2. Meeker et al., "Consensus."
3. Department of Health, "Prevalence."
4. Shekelle et al., "Congruence."
5. Bronfort et al., "Efficacy."
6. Meade et al., "Randomised."
7. Croft et al., "Outcome."
8. Coulter and Shekelle, "IV. Supply."
9. Richard et al., "Expenditures."
10. Giles and Muller, "Chronic."
11. Hondras et al., "Randomized."
12. Bishop et al., "Chiropractic."
13. Little et al., "General."
14. Bonebrake et al., "Treatment for carpal tunnel syndrome: evaluation"; Bonebrake et al., "Treatment for carpal tunnel syndrome: results."
15. Arslan and Celiker, "Comparison"; Winters et al., "Comparison."
16. Boline et al., "Spinal."

17. Nelson et al., "Efficacy."
18. Tuchin, Pollard, and Bonello, "Randomized."
19. Turk and Ratkolb, "Mobilization."
20. Jensen, Nielsen, and Vosmar, "Open study."
21. McCrory, *Evidence Report.*
22. Kokjohn et al., "Effect."
23. Fallon, "Role"; Fallon and Edelman, "Chiropractic care."
24. Vernon, Humphreys, and Hagino, "Chronic."

10. ACUPUNCTURE AND QIGONG

1. Mayer, Price, and Rafii, "Antagonism"; Pomeranz and Chiu, "Naloxone."
2. Pomeranz and Bibic, "Electroacupuncture"; Pomeranz and Chiu, "Naloxone."
3. "Acupuncture."
4. Lao et al., "Evaluation."
5. Habek et al., "Efficacy"; Liu et al., "Immediate."
6. Vincent, "Controlled"; Linde et al., "Acupuncture."
7. Micozzi, *Celestial*, 65–78.

11. VITAMINS, NUTRITIONAL FOODS, AND HERBS

1. USA Food and Beverage Market Study, 2013. Switzerland Global Enterprise. www.s-ge.com/sites/default/files/private_files/BBK_Foodstudie_USA _June%202013_0.pdf; see also Eisenberg, Davis, and Ettner, "Trends"; Johnson, "Herbal."
2. Fugh-Berman, "Herb-drug"; Fugh-Berman and Cott, "Dietary."
3. Shils, "Nutrition."
4. Kim, "Role." See also Pericleous, Mandair, and Caplin, "Diet."
5. Morris et al., "Dietary." See also Malouf, Grimley, and Areosa, "Folic."
6. Jacobson, Plancher, and Kleinman, "Vitamin B6."
7. Hammond et al., "Nutritional."
8. Maizels, Blumenfeld, and Burchette, "Combination."
9. Smedby et al., "Ultraviolet."
10. Wilkins et al., "Vitamin D"; Khamba et al., "Effectiveness."
11. Morley, "Dementia"; Veugelers and Ekwaru, "Statistical"; Heaney et al., "Letter."
12. Dysken et al., "Effect."
13. Tütüncü, Bayraktar, and Varli, "Reversal"; Bansal, Kalita, and Misra, "Diabetic."
14. Cotter and O'Keeffe, "Restless."
15. O'Keeffe, Gavin, and Lavan, "Iron."
16. Ziegler and Gries, "Alpha-lipoic"; Singh and Jialal, "Alpha-lipoic"; Higdon, "Lipoic acid."

17. Vamvakas et al., "Alcohol"; Gullestad et al., "Magnesium"; Rivlin, "Magnesium"; Swaminathan, "Hypo-hypermagnesaemia."
18. Bigal et al., "Intravenous"; Bigal et al., "Migraine"; Blumenthal, *ABC*; Pfaffenrath et al., "Magnesium"; Mauskop and Varughese, "Why."
19. Peikert, Wilimzig, and Köhne-Volland, "Prophylaxis"; Mauskop and Altura, "Role"; Mauskop, Altura, and Altura, "Serum"; Wang et al., "Oral."
20. Sherwood et al., "Magnesium"; Rosenstein et al., "Magnesium"; Bigal et al., "Intravenous"; Bigal et al., "Migraine."
21. Wilson and Murphy, "Herbal and dietary."
22. Facchinetti et al., "Magnesium."
23. Yagi et al., "Role"; Tupe and Chiplonkar, "Zinc."
24. Aiba et al., "Effect of zinc sulfate"; Welge-Lüssen, "Re-establishment."
25. Najafizade et al., "Preventive."
26. Rubin, "New"; Mynott et al., "Bromelain"; Kerkhoffs et al., "Double blind"; Kamenícek, Holán, and Franĕk, "Systemic"; Braun, Schneider, and Beuth, "Therapeutic."
27. Logan, "Omega-3"; Robinson, Ijioma, and Harris, "Omega-3."
28. Ko et al., "Omega-3"; Heller et al., "Omega-3."
29. Mulrow et al., "Garlic."
30. Rahman and Lowe, "Aged."
31. Aragon et al., "Probiotic."
32. Biswal et al., "Effect"; Mishra, *Rheumatoid,* 10; Mishra and Singh, "Scientific."
33. Kimmatkar et al., "Efficacy."
34. Deal, Schnitzer, and Lipstein, "Treatment."
35. Weinmann et al., "Effects."
36. Van Dongen et al., "Ginkgo."
37. Kanowski et al., "Proof."
38. Hashiguchi et al., "Meta-analysis."
39. Oken, Storzbach, and Kaye, "Efficacy."
40. Von Boetticher, "Ginkgo biloba."
41. Dubreuil, "Therapeutic."
42. Hoffmann et al., "Ginkgo."
43. Hamann, "Physikalische."
44. Volz and Kieser, "Kava-kava"; Geier and Konstantinowicz, "Kava."
45. Pittler and Ernst, "Efficacy."
46. Kinzler, Kromer, and Lehmann, "Wirksamkeit."
47. Gruenwald and Skrabal, "Kava."
48. Ji et al., "Flavokawain B."
49. Tillu et al., "Resveratrol."
50. Dipti, Tillu, and Melemedjian, "Resveratrol."

51. Goldbach-Mansky et al., "Comparison."
52. Aggarwal and Harikumar, "Potential."
53. "Valerian root," in Blumenthal, Goldberg, and Brinckmann, *Herbal Medicine*, 394–400.
54. Lindahl and Lindwall, "Double blind."

12. ESSENTIAL OILS AND AROMATHERAPY

1. Valnet, *Practice.*
2. Tisserand, *Art.*
3. Steele, "Anthropology."
4. Stoddart, "Human odour."
5. Valnet, *Practice.*
6. Tisserand, *Art.*
7. Arcier, *Aromatherapy.*
8. Williams, "Lecture."
9. Arcier, *Aromatherapy.*
10. Steele, "Anthropology."
11. Franchomme and Pénoël, *L'aromatherapie.*
12. Maury, *Secret.*
13. Holmes, *Clinical*; Holmes, *Energetics*; Miller and Miller, *Ayurveda.*
14. Franchomme and Pénoël, *L'aromatherapie.*
15. Ibid.
16. Valnet, *Practice.*
17. Hotchkiss, "How thin."
18. Jäger et al., "Percutaneous."
19. Ibid.
20. Bronough, "In vivo"; Collins et al., "Some observations."
21. Tisserand and Young, *Essential Oil.*
22. Buchbauer et al., "Aromatherapy."
23. Stevensen, "Psychophysiological."
24. Madison, "Psychophysiological."
25. Longworth, "Psychophysiological."
26. Bauer and Dracup, "Physiologic."
27. Dunn, "Report."
28. Freud, *Civilization.*
29. Shepherd, *Neurobiology.*
30. Hardy, "Sweet"; Stevensen, "Psychophysiological."
31. Lorenzetti et al., "Myrcene."
32. Fellowes, Barnes, and Wilkinson, "Aromatherapy."
33. Thorgrimsen et al., "Aromatherapy."
34. Smith et al., "Complementary."

35. Egan et al., "Availability."

36. Buchbauer et al., "Aromatherapy."

37. Torii et al., "Contingent."

38. Stevensen, "Psychophysiological."

39. Buckle, "Aromatherapy"; Lawless, *Illustrated*; Tisserand and Balacs, *Essential*; Kim et al., "Effect."

40. Dunn, "Report."

41. Wilkinson et al., "Evaluation."

42. Hardy, "Sweet."

Bibliography

Abbot, N. C., E. F. Harkness, C. Stevinson, F. P. Marshall, D. A. Conn, and E. Ernst. "Spiritual Healing as a Therapy for Chronic Pain: A Randomized, Clinical Trial." *Int Assoc Study Pain* 91 (2001): 79–89.

"Acupuncture." NIH Consensus Statement Online 15, no. 5 (Nov 3–5, 1997): 1–34.

Aggarwal, B. B., and K. B. Harikumar. "Potential Therapeutic Effects of Curcumin, the Anti-inflammatory Agent, against Neurodegenerative, Cardiovascular, Pulmonary, Metabolic, Autoimmune and Neoplastic Diseases." *Int J Biochem Cell Biol* 41, no. 1 (2009): 40–59. doi: 10.1016/j.biocel.2008.06.010.

Aiba, T., M. Sugiura, J. Mori, et al. "Effect of Zinc Sulfate on Sensorineural Olfactory Disorder." *Acta Otolaryngol* suppl. (Stockh) 538 (1998): 202–4.

American Masssage Therapy Association (AMTA). "Industry Fact Sheet." February 2016. www.amtamassage.org/infocenter/economic_industry-fact-sheet.html.

———. "Living Right: Talking to Your Physician about Massage—Fact Sheet." December 6, 2011. www.amtamassage.org/uploads/cms/documents/livingrightlr.pdf.

———. "Use of Massage Therapy in Hospitals Up 30 Percent." May 24, 2006. www.amtamassage.org/articles/2/PressRelease/detail/2105.

Appelboom, T., N. Maes, and A. Albert. "A New Curcuma Extract (Flexofytol) in Osteoarthritis: Results from a Belgian Real-Life Experience." *Open Rheumatol J* 8 (Oct 17, 2014): 77–81.

Aragon, G., D. B. Graham, M. Borum, and D. B. Doman. "Probiotic Therapy for Irritable Bowel Syndrome." *Gastroenterol Hepatol* 6, no. 1 (Jan 2010): 39–44. PMCID: PMC2886445.

Arcier, Micheline. *Aromatherapy*. London: Hamlyn, 1990.

Arora, R., A. Kuhad, I. P. Kaur, K. Chopra. "Curcumin Loaded Solid Lipid Nanoparticles Ameliorate Adjuvant-Induced Arthritis in Rats." *Eur J Pain* 19, no. 7 (2015): 940–52.

Arslan, S., and R. Celiker. "Comparison of the Efficacy of Local Corticosteroid Injection and Physical Therapy for the Treatment of Adhesive Capsulitis." *Rheumatol Int* 21 (2001): 20–23.

Baars, Bernard J., and Nicole M. Gage. *Cognition, Brain and Consciousness.* Burlington, Mass.: Elsevier, 2010.

Bansal, V., J. Kalita, and U. K. Misra. "Diabetic Neuropathy." *Postgraduate Med J* 82, no. 964 (2006): 95–100. doi: 10.1136/pgmj.2005.036137.

Banth, S., and M. Didehdar Ardebil. "Effectiveness of Mindfulness Meditation on Pain and Quality of Life of Patients with Chronic Low Back Pain." *Int J Yoga* 8, no. 2 (Jul–Dec 2015): 128–33.

Barber, J., and J. Gitelson. "Cancer Pain: Psychological Management Using Hypnosis." *Ca Cancer J Clin* 30 (1980): 130–36.

Barber, Theodore X. *Hypnosis: A Scientific Approach.* Oxford, England: Van Nostrand Reinhold, 1969.

Barber, T. X., H. Chauncey, and R. Winer. "Effect of Hypnotic and Nonhypnotic Suggestions on Parotid Gland Response to Gustatory Stimuli." *Psychosom Med* 26 (1964): 374–80.

Barlow, David H., and V. Mark Durand. *Abnormal Psychology: An Integrative Approach,* 7th ed. Stamford, Conn.: Cengage Learning, 2014.

Bartlett, S. J., S. Haaz, C. Mill, S. Bernatsky, and C. O. Bingham. "Yoga in Rheumatic Diseases." *Current Rheumat Rep* 15, no. 12 (2013): 387. doi: 10.1007/s11926-013-0387-2.

Bauer, W. C., and K. A. Dracup. "Physiologic Effects of Back Massage in Patients with Acute Myocardial Infarction." *Focus Crit Care* 14, no. 6 (1987): 42–46.

Bay, R., and F. Bay. "Combined Therapy Using Acupressure Therapy, HypnoTherapy, and Transcendental Meditation versus Placebo in Type 2 Diabetes." *J Acupunct Meridian Stud* 4, no. 3 (Sep 2011): 183–86. www.ncbi.nlm.nih.gov/pubmed/21981869.

Bechtel, William, and Robert C. Richardson. "Vitalism." In *Routledge Encyclopedia of Philosophy,* edited by E. Craig. London: Routledge, 1998.

Belcaro, G., M. Dugall, R. Luzzi, et al. "Management of Osteoarthritis (OA) with the Pharma-Standard Supplement Flexiqule (Boswellia): A 12 Week Registry." *Minerva Gastroenterol Dietol* (Oct 22, 2015 epub ahead of print).

Beneliyahu, D. J. "Magnetic Resonance Imaging and Clinical Follow-Up: Study of 27 Patients Receiving Chiropractic Care for Cervical and Lumbar Disc Herniations." *J Manipulative Physiol Ther* 19, no. 9 (1996): 597–606.

Bennett, H. L. "A Comparison of Audiotaped Preparations for Surgery: Evaluation and Outcomes." Paper presented at the annual meeting of the

Society for Clinical and Experimental Hypnosis. Tampa, Fla., 1996.

Benson, Herbert. "The Relaxation Response." In *Mind-Body Medicine: How to Use Your Mind for Better Health,* edited by David Goleman and Joel Gunn, 233–57. Yonkers, N.Y.: Consumer Reports, 1998.

Benson, H., R. F. Steinert, M. M. Greenwood, H. M. Klemchuk, and N. H. Peterson. "Continuous Measurement of Oxygen Consumption and Carbon Dioxide Elimination during a Wakeful Hypometabolic State." *J Human Stress* 1, no. 1 (Mar 1975): 37–44.

Bhasin, M. K., J. A. Dusek, B. H. Chang, M. G. Joseph, J. W. Denninger, G. L. Fricchione, H. Benson, and T. A. Libermann. "Relaxation Response Induces Temporal Transcriptome Changes in Energy Metabolism, Insulin Secretion and Inflammatory Pathways." *Plos ONE* 8, no. 5 (2013): E62817.

Bigal, M. E., C. A. Bordini, F. D. Sheftell, J. G. Speciali, and J. O. M. Bigal. "Migraine with Aura Versus Migraine without Aura: Pain Intensity and Associated Symptom Intensities after Placebo." *Headache: J Head and Face Pain* 42 (2002): 872–77. doi:10.1046/j.1526-4610.2002.02205.x.

Bigal, M. E., C. A. Bordini, S. J. Tepper, et al. "Intravenous Magnesium Sulfate in the Acute Treatment of Migraine with and without Aura." *Cephalalgia* 22 (2002): 345–440.

Bishop, P. B., J. A. Quon, C. G. Fisher, and M. F. S. Dvorak. "The Chiropractic Hospital-Based Interventions Research Outcomes (CHIRO) Study: A Randomized Controlled Trial on the Effectiveness of Clinical Practice Guidelines in the Medical and Chiropractic Management of Patients with Acute Mechanical Low Back Pain." *Spine J* 10, no. 12 (2010): 1055–64.

Biswal, B. M., S. A. Sulaiman, H. C. Ismail, H. Zakaria, and K. L. Musa. "Effect of Withania somnifera (Ashwagandha) on the Development of Chemotherapy-Induced Fatigue and Quality of Life in Breast Cancer Patients." *Integr Cancer Ther* 12, no. 4 (Jul 2013): 312–22. Epub Nov 9, 2012. doi: 10.1177/1534735412464551.

Blakeslee, Sandra, Stephen L. Macknik, and Susana Martinez-Conde. *Sleights of Mind: What the Neuroscience of Magic Reveals about Our Brains.* Great Britain: Clays, Bungay, Suffolk, 2011.

Blumenthal, Mark. *The ABC Clinical Guide to Herbs.* Austin, Tex.: American Botanical Council, 2003.

Blumenthal, Mark, Alicia Goldberg, and Josef Brinckmann. *Herbal Medicine: Expanded Commission E Monographs.* Newton, Mass.: Integrative Medicine Communications, 2000.

Boline, P. D., K. Kassak, G. Bronfort, C. Nelson, and A. V. Anderson. "Spinal Manipulation versus Amitriptyline for the Treatment of Chronic Tension-Type Headaches: A Randomized Clinical Trial." *J Manipulative Physiol Ther* 18, no. 3 (1995): 148–54.

Bonebrake, A. R., J. E. Fernandez, J. B. Dahalan, and R. J. Marley. "A Treatment for Carpal Tunnel Syndrome: Results of a Follow-Up Study." *J Manipulative Physiol Ther* 16, no. 3 (1993): 125–39.

Bonebrake, A. R., J. E. Fernandez, R. J. Marley, J. B. Dahalan, and K. J. Kilmer. "A Treatment for Carpal Tunnel Syndrome: Evaluation of Objective and Subjective Measures." *J Manipulative Physiol Ther* 13, no. 9 (1990): 507–20.

Braud, W. G. "Human Interconnectedness: Research Indications." *ReVision* 14 (1992): 140–48.

Braun, J. M., B. Schneider, and H. J. Beuth. "Therapeutic Use, Efficiency and Safety of the Proteolytic Pineapple Enzyme Bromelain-POS in Children with Acute Sinusitis in Germany." *In Vivo* 19, no. 2 (Mar–Apr 2005): 417–21.

Brody, Jane E. "Let the Mind Help Tame an Irritable Bowel." *New York Times,* Sep 1, 2008. www.nytimes.com/2008/09/02/health/02brod.html.

Bronfort, G., M. Haas, R. L. Evans, and L. M. Bouter. "Efficacy of Spinal Manipulation and Mobilization for Low Back Pain and Neck Pain: A Systematic Review and Best Evidence Synthesis." *Spine J* 4, no. 3 (2004): 335–56.

Bronough, R. L. "In Vivo Percutaneous Absorption of Fragrance Ingredients in Rhesus Monkeys and Humans." *Food Chem Toxicol* 28, no. 5 (1990): 369–74.

Brooks, J. S., and T. Scarano. "Transcendental Meditation in the Treatment of Post-Vietnam Adjustment." *J Counseling and Development* 64 (1985): 212–15. doi:10.1002/j.1556-6676.1985.tb01078.x.

Buchbauer, G., L. Jirovetz, W. Jäger, H. Dietrich, and C. Plank. "Aromatherapy: Evidence for Sedative Effects of the Essential Oil of Lavender after inhalation." *Z Naturforsch* 46 (1991): 1067–72.

Buckle, J. "Aromatherapy: Does It Matter Which Lavender Oil Is Used?" *Nurs Times* 89, no. 20 (1993): 32–35.

Byrd, R. C. "Positive Therapeutic Effects of Intercessory Prayer in a Coronary Care Unit Population." *Southern Med J* 81, no. 7 (1988): 826–29.

Carlson, L. E., Z. Ursuliak, E. Goodey, M. Angen, and M. Speca. "The Effects of a Mindfulness Meditation-Based Stress Reduction Program on Mood and Symptoms of Stress in Cancer Outpatients: 6-Month Follow-Up." *Support Care Cancer* 9, no. 2 (Mar 2001): 112–23.

Chaitow, Leon. *Muscle Energy Techniques,* 4th ed. New York: Churchill Livingstone, 2013.

Chaitow, Leon, and Judith DeLany. *The Upper Body.* Vol. 1 of *Clinical Applications of Neuromuscular Techniques.* New York: Churchill Livingstone, 2000.

———. *The Lower Body.* Vol. 2 of *Clinical Application of Neuromuscular Techniques.* New York: Churchill Livingstone, 2011.

Chang, B. H., D. Jones, A. Hendricks, U. Boehmer, J. S. Locastro, and M. Slawsky. "Relaxation Response for Veterans Affairs Patients with Congestive Heart Failure: Results from a Qualitative Study within a Clinical Trial." *Prev Cardiol* 7, no. 2 (Spring 2004): 64–70.

Chaya, M. S., and H. R. Nagendra. "Long-Term Effect of Yogic Practices on Diurnal Metabolic Rates of Healthy Subjects." *Int J Yoga* 1, no. 1 (Jan–Jun 2008): 27–32. doi: 10.4103/0973-6131.36761. PMCID: PMC3144606.

Collins, A. J., L. J. Notarianni, E. F. Ring, and M. P Seed. "Some Observations on the Pharmacology of 'Deep-Heat,' A Topical Rubefacient." *Ann Rheum Dis* 43, no. 3 (1984): 411–15.

Cooper, M. J., and M. M. Aygen. "The Effect of Meditation on Serum Cholesterol and Blood Pressure." *J Israel Med Assoc* 95 (1978): 1–2.

Cotter, P. E., and S. T. O'Keeffe. "Restless Leg Syndrome: Is It a Real Problem? *Ther Clin Risk Manag* 2, no. 4 (2006): 465–75.

Coulter, Ian D., and Paul G. Shekelle. "IV. Supply, Distribution, and Utilization of Chiropractors in the United States." In *Chiropractic in the United States: Training, Practice, and Research,* edited by Daniel C. Cherkin and Robert D. Mootz. Agency for Health Care Policy and Research, December 1997. www .sonic.net/jet/chiroinus2.pdf.

Croft, P. R., G. J. Macfarlane, A. C. Papageorgiou, E. Thomas, and A. J. Silman. "Outcome of Low Back Pain in General Practice: A Prospective Study." *Brit Med J* 316, no. 7141 (1998): 1356–59.

Cyna, A. M. "Hypno-Analgesia for a Labouring Parturient with Contra-Indications to Central Neuraxial Block." *Anaesthesia* 58 (2003): 101–2.

Cyna, A. M., G. L. Mcauliffe, and M. I. Andrew. "Hypnosis for Pain Relief in Labor and Childbirth: A Systematic Review." *Brit J Anesth* 93, no. 4 (2004): 505–11.

Danucalov, M. A., R. S. Simões, E. H. Kozasa, and J. R. Leite. "Cardiorespiratory and Metabolic Changes during Yoga Sessions: The Effects of Respiratory Exercises and Meditation Practices." *Appl Psychophysiol Biofeedback* 33, no. 2 (Jun 2008): 77–81. Epub Mar 4, 2008. doi: 10.1007/s10484-008-9053-2.

Deal, C. L., T. J. Schnitzer, and E. Lipstein. "Treatment of Arthritis with Topical Capsaicin: A Double-Blind Trial." *Clin Ther* 13, no. 3 (1991): 383–95.

DeBenedittis, G., A. A. Panerai, and M. A. Villamira. "Effects of Hypnotic Analgesia and Hypnotizability on Experimental Ischemic Pain." *Int J Clin Exp Hypn* 37, no. 1 (Jan. 1989): 55–69.

Department of Health. "The Prevalence of Back Pain in Great Britain in 1998." London: Government Statistical Service, 1999.

Desikachar, K., L. Bragdon, and C. Bossart. "The Yoga of Healing: Exploring Yoga's Holistic Model for Health and Well-Being." *Int J Yoga Ther* 15 (2005): 17–39.

Dipti, V., O. K. Tillu, and M. N. Melemedjian. "Resveratrol Engages AMPK to Attenuate ERK and mTOR Signaling in Sensory Neurons and Inhibits Incision-Induced Acute and Chronic Pain." *Mol Pain* 8, no. 5 (2012). doi:10.1186/1744-8069-8-5.

Donesky-Cuenco, D., H. Q. Nguyen, S. Paul, and V. Carrieri-Kohlman. "Yoga Therapy Decreases Dyspnea-Related Distress and Improves Functional Performance in People with Chronic Obstructive Pulmonary Disease: A Pilot Study." *J Altern Complement Med* 15, no. 3 (Mar 2009): 225–34. doi: 10.1089/acm.2008.0389. PMCID: PMC3051406. NIHMSID: NIHMS267868.

Donoyama, N., T. Munakata, and M. Shibasaki. "Effects of Anma Therapy (Traditional Japanese Massage) on Body and Mind." *J Bodyw Mov Ther* 14, no. 1 (Jan 2010): 55–64. doi: 10.1016/j.jbmt.2008.06.007.

Donoyama, N., T. Satoh, and T. Hamano. "Effects of Anma Therapy (Traditional Japanese Massage) for Gynecological Cancer Survivors: Study Protocol for a Randomized Controlled Trial." *Trials* 14 (2013): 233. doi: 10.1186/1745-6215-14-233.

Donoyama, N., T. Satoh, T. Hamano, N. Ohkoshi, and M. Onuki. "Physical Effects of Anma Therapy (Japanese Massage) for Gynecologic Cancer Survivors: A Randomized Controlled Trial." *Gynecol Oncol* 142, no. 3 (Sep 2016): 531–38. doi: 10.1016/j.ygyno.2016.06.022.

Draucker, C. B., A. F. Jacobson, W. A. Umberger, et al. "Acceptability of a Guided Imagery Intervention for Persons Undergoing a Total Knee Replacement." *Orthop Nurs* 34, no. 6 (Nov–Dec 2015): 356–64.

Dubreuil, C. "Therapeutic Trial in Acute Cochlear Deafness: A Comparative Study of Ginkgo Biloba Extract and Nicergoline." *Presse Med* 15 (1986): 1559–61.

Dunn, B. R., J. A. Hartigan, and W. L. Mikulas. "Concentration and Mindfulness Meditations: Unique Forms of Consciousness?" *Appl Psychophysiol Biofeedback* 24, no. 3 (Sep 1999): 147–65.

Dunn, C. "A Report on a Randomized Controlled Trial to Evaluate the Use of Massage and Aromatherapy in an Intensive Care Unit." Unpublished paper. Battle Hospital, Reading, England, 1992.

Dysken, M. W., M. Sano, S. Asthana, et al. "Effect of Vitamin E and Memantine on Functional Decline in Alzheimer Disease: The TEAM-AD VA Cooperative Randomized Trial." *J Am Med Assoc* 311, no. 1 (2014): 33–44. doi:10.1001/jama.2013.282834.

Egan, B., H. Gage, J. Hood, K. Poole, C. Mcdowell, and L. Storey. "Availability of Complementary and Alternative Medicine for People with Cancer in the British National Health Service: Results of a National Survey." *Complement Ther Clin Practice* 18, no. 2 (2012): 75–80.

Ehrlich, S. D. "Hypnotherapy." University of Maryland Medical Center, 2011. http://umm.edu/health/medical/altmed/treatment/hypnotherapy.

Eisenberg, D. M., R. B. Davis, and S. L. Ettner. "Trends in Alternative Medicine Use in the United States, 1990–1997: Results of a Follow-Up National Survey." *J Am Med Assoc* 280 (1998): 1569–75.

Ellis, M. R., D. C. Vinson, and B. J. Ewigman. "Addressing Spiritual Concerns of Patients: Family Physicians' Attitudes and Practices." *Fam Pract* 48, no. 2 (Feb 1999): 105–9.

Enqvist, B., and K. Fisher. "Preoperative Hypnotic Techniques Reduce Consumption of Analgesics after Surgical Removal of Third Mandibular Molars: A Brief Communication." *Int J Clin Exp Hypn* 45 (1997): 102–8.

Enqvist, B., L. Von Konow, and H. Bystedt. "Stress Reduction, Preoperative Hypnosis and Perioperative Suggestions in Maxillo-Facial Surgery." *Stress Med* 11 (1995): 229–33.

Esch, T., G. B. Stefano, G. L. Fricchione, and H. Benson. "Stress in Cardiovascular Diseases." *Med Science Monitor* 8, no. 5 (2002): RA93–RA101.

Espi-Lopez, G. V., R. Zurriaga-Llorens, L. Monzani, and D. Falla. "The Effect of Manipulation Plus Massage Therapy versus Massage Therapy Alone in People with Tention-Type Headache: A Randomized Controlled Clinical Trial." *Eur J Phys Rehabil Med* (Mar 18 2016; epub ahead of print).

Facchinetti, F. L., G. Sances, P. Borella, A. R. Genazzani, and G. Nappi. "Magnesium Prophylaxis of Menstrual Migraine: Effects of Iintracellular Magnesium." *Headache* 31 (1991): 298–301.

Fallon, J. "The Role of the Chiropractic Adjustment in the Care and Treatment of 332 Children with Otitis Media." *J Clin Chiropr Ped* 2, no. 2 (1997): 167–83.

Fallon, J., and M. J. Edelman. "Chiropractic Care of 401 Children with Otitis Media: A Pilot Study." *Altern Ther Health Med* 4, no. 2 (1998): 93.

Fellowes, D., K. Barnes, and S. Wilkinson. "Aromatherapy and Massage for Symptom Relief in Patients with Cancer." *Cochrane Database Syst Rev* 3 (2004).

Feuerstein, George. "The History and Literature of Patanjala-Yoga." Chapter 9 in *The Yoga Tradition: Its History, Literature, Philosophy, and Practice.* Prescott, Ariz.: Hohm Press, 2001.

Field, T. M. "Massage Therapy Effect." *Am Psychol* 53 (1998): 1270–81.

Franchomme, Pierre, and Daniel Pénoël. *L'aromatherapie exactement.* Limoges, France: Roger Jallois, 1990.

Freud, Sigmund. *Civilization and Its Discontents.* Vol. 21 of *The Complete Psychological Works.* Edited by James Strachy. London: Hogath Press, 1930.

Fugh-Berman, A. "Herb-Drug Interactions." *Lancet* 355 (2000): 134–38.

Fugh-Berman, A., and J. Cott. "Dietary Supplements and Natural Products as Psychotherapeutic Agents." *Psychosom Med* 61 (1999): 712–28.

Ganis, G., W. L. Thompson, and S. M. Kosslyn. "Brain Areas Underlying Visual Mental Imagery and Visual Perception: An FMRI Study." *Brain Res Cogn Brain Res* 20, no. 2 (Jul 2004): 226–41. www.ncbi.nlm.nih.gov /pubmed/15183394.

Gehl, Jennifer T., and Marc Micozzi. *The Science of Planetary Signatures in Medicine.* Rochester, Vt.: Healing Arts Press, 2017.

Geier, F. P., and T. Konstantinowicz. "Kava Treatment in Patients with Anxiety." *Phytother Res* 18 (2004): 297–300. doi:10.1002/ptr.1422.

Ghoneim, M. M., R. I. Block, D. S. Sarasin, C. S. Davis, and J. N. Marchman. "Tape-Recorded Hypnosis Instructions as Adjuvant in the Care of Patients Scheduled for Third Molar Surgery." *Anesth Analg* 90 (2000): 64.

Giles, L. G., and R. Muller. "Chronic Spinal Pain: A Randomized Clinical Trial Comparing Medication, Acupuncture, and Spinal Manipulation." *Spine* 28, no. 14 (2003): 1490–502.

Goldbach-Mansky, R., M. Wilson, R. Fleischmann et al. "Comparison of Tripterygium wilfordii Hook F versus Sulfasalazine in the Treatment of Rheumatoid Arthritis: A Randomized Trial." *Ann Intern Med* 151, no. 4 (2009): 229–40.

Goldberg, Michelle. *The Goddess Pose: The Audacious Life of Indra Devi, the Woman Who Helped Bring Yoga to the West.* New York: Vintage, 2016.

Goldsmith, Margaret. *Franz Anton Mesmer: A History of Mesmerism.* Garden City, N.Y.: Doubleday, Doran, and Company, 1934.

Gordon, D. "The Fresh Face of Hypnosis: An Old Practice Finds New Uses." *Better Homes and Gardens,* Feb 2004.

Gosline, A. "Hypnosis Really Changes Your Mind." *New Scientist* 9–10 (2004).

Gothe, N. P., A. F. Kramer, and E. McAuley. "The Effects of an 8-Week Hatha Yoga Intervention on Executive Function in Older Adults." *J Gerontol A Biol Sci Med Sci* 69, no. 9 (Sep 2014): 1109–16. www.ncbi.nlm.nih.gov /pubmed/25024234.

Graci, Gina, and Kathy Sexton-Radek. "Treating Sleep Disorders Using Cognitive Behavior Therapy and Hypnosis." In *The Clinical Use of Hypnosis in Cognitive Behavior Therapy: A Practitioner's Casebook*, edited by Robin A. Chapman, 296. New York: Springer, 2006.

Green, Elmer, and Alyce Green. *Beyond Biofeedback.* New York: Knoll Publishing, 1977.

Gruenwald, J., and J. Skrabal. "Kava Ban Highly Questionable: Brief Summary of the Main Scientific Findings Presented in the 'In Depth Investigation on European Union Member States Market Restrictions on Kava Products.'" *Sem Integrative Med* 1, no. 4 (2003): 199–210.

Gullestad, L., L. O. Dolva, A. Waage, D. Falch, H. Fagerthun, and J. Kjekshus.

"Magnesium Deficiency Diagnosed by an Intravenous Loading Test." *Scand J Clin Lab Invest* 52 (1992): 245–53.

Gura, S. T. "Yoga for Stress Reduction and Injury Prevention at Work." *Work* 19 (2002): 3–7.

Habek, D., J. Cerkez Habek, M. Bobic-Vukovic, and B. Vujic. "Efficacy of Acupuncture for the Treatment of Primary Dymenorrheal." *Gynakol Geburtshilfliche Rundsch* 43, no. 4 (Oct 2003): 250–53.

Hamann, K. F. "Physikalische Therapie des vestibulären Schwindels in Verbindung mit Ginkgo-biloba-Extrakt." *Therapiewoche* 35 (1985): 4586–90.

Hammond, A. N., Y. Wang, M. Dimachkie, and R. Barohn. "Nutritional Neuropathies." *Neurologic Clinics* 31, no. 2 (2013): 477–89. doi: 10.1016/j.ncl.2013.02.002.

Hardy, M. "Sweet Scented Dreams." *Int J Aromather* 3, no. 1 (1991): 12–13.

Harris, W. S., M. Gowda, J. W. Kolb, et al. "A Randomized, Controlled Trial of the Effects of Remote, Intercessory Prayer on Outcomes in Patients Admitted to the Coronary Care Unit." *Archives Intern Med* 159, no. 19 (1999): 2273–78.

Hartmann, Ernest. *Dreams and Nightmares: The Origin and Meaning of Dreams.* New York: Plenum Press, 1998.

Harvard Health Publications. "Depression and Pain." Harvard Medical School, June 2009. www.health.harvard.edu/mind-and-mood/depression_and_pain.

Hashiguchi, M., Y. Ohta, M. Shimizu, J. Maruyama, and M. Mochizuki. "Meta-Analysis of the Efficacy and Safety of Ginkgo biloba Extract for the Treatment of Dementia." *J Pharm Health Care Sci* 1 (Apr 2015): 14. doi: 10.1186/s40780-015-0014-7.

Häuser, W., C. Bartram, E. Bartram-Wunn, and T. Tölle. "Systematic Review: Adverse Events Attributable to Nocebo in Randomised Controlled Drug Trials in Fibromyalgia Syndrome and Painful Diabetic Peripheral Neuropathy." *Clin J Pain* 28 (2012): 437–51.

Häuser, W., E. Hansen, and P. Enck. "Nocebo Phenomena in Medicine: Their Relevance in Everyday Clinical Practice." *Deutsches Ärzteblatt Int* 109, no. 26 (2012): 459–65.

Heaney, R., C. Garland, C. Baggerly, C. French, and E. Gorham. "Letter to Veugelers, P.J. and Ekwaru, J.P., A Statistical Error in the Estimation of the Recommended Dietary Allowance for Vitamin D." *Nutrients* 7, no. 3 (March 2015): 1688–90. www.mdpi.com/2072-6643/7/3/1688.

Heath, I. "Waste and Harm in the Treatment of Hypertension." *J Am Med Assoc Intern Med* 173, no. 11 (2013): 956–57.

Heller, A. R., S. Rössler, R. J. Litz, et al. "Omega-3 Fatty Acids Improve the Diagnosis-Related Clinical Outcome." *Crit Care Med* 34, no. 4 (Apr 2006): 972–79.

Herbert, Nick. *Quantum Reality: Beyond the New Physics.* New York: Anchor Books, 1985.

Hewett, Z. L., L. B. Ransdell, Y. Gao, L. M. Petlichkoff, and S. M. Lucas. "An Examination of the Effectiveness of an 8-Week Bikram Yoga Program on Mindfulness, Perceived Stress, and Physical Fitness." Boise State University ScholarWorks, 2011. http://scholarworks.boisestate.edu/cgi/viewcontent.cgi ?article=1089&context=kinesiology_facpubs.

Higdon, J. "Lipoic Acid." Linus Pauling Institute Micronutrient Information Center, 2002. http://lpi.oregonstate.edu/infocenter/othernuts/la/.

Hill, C. L., L. M. March, D. Aitken, et al. "Fish Oil in Knee Osteoarthritis: A Randomized Clinical Trial of Low Dose versus High Dose." *Ann Rheum Dis* 75, no. 1 (Jan 2016): 23–29.

Hoffmann, F., C. Beck, A. Schutz, and P. Offermann. "Ginkgo Extract EGB 761 (Tebonin)/HAES versus Naftidrofuryl (Dusodril)/HAES: A Randomized Study of Therapy of Sudden Deafness." *Laryngorhinootologie* 73 (1994): 149–52. [Article in German.]

Holmes, Peter. *Clinical Aromatherapy.* Cotati, Calif.: Tigerlily Press, 2008.

———. *The Energetics of Western Herbs,* 4th ed. 2 vols. Boulder, Colo.: Snow Lotus Press, 2007.

Hondras, M. A., C. R. Long, Y. Cao, R. M. Rowell, and W. C. Meeker. "A Randomized Controlled Trial Comparing 2 Types of Spinal Manipulation and Minimal Conservative Medical Care for Adults 55 Years and Older with Subacute or Chronic Low Back Pain." *J Manipulative Physiol Ther* 32, no. 5 (Jun 2009): 330–43.

Hotchkiss, S. "How Thin Is Your Skin?" *New Scientist* 141, no. 1910 (1994): 24–27.

Jacobson, M. D., K. D. Plancher, and W. B. Kleinman. "Vitamin B6 (Pyridoxine) Therapy for Carpal Tunnel Syndrome." *Hand Clin* 12 (1996): 253–57.

Jäger, W., G. Buckbauer, L. Jirovetz, and M. Fritzer. "Percutaneous Absorption of Lavender Oil from a Massage Oil." *J Soc Cosmetic Chem* 43 (1992): 49–54.

Jahn, Robert G., and Brenda J. Dunne. "Precognitive Remote Perception." In *Margins of Reality: The Role of Consciousness in the Physical World,* 149–91. New York: Harcourt Brace Jovanovich, 1987.

Jaju, D. S., M. B. Dikshit, J. Balaji, J. George, S. Rizvi, and O. Al-Rawas. "Effects of Pranayam Breathing on Respiratory Pressures and Sympathovagal Balance of Patients with Chronic Airflow Limitation and in Control Subjects." *Sultan Qaboos Univ Med J* 11, no. 2 (May 2011): 221–29. Published online May 15, 2011. PMCID: PMC3121027.

Jawer, Michael, and Marc Miccozi. *Spiritual Anatomy of Emotion.* Rochester, Vt.: Park Street Press, 2009.

———. *Your Emotional Type.* Rochester, Vt.: Healing Arts Press, 2011.

Jensen, O. K., F. F. Nielsen, and L. Vosmar. "An Open Study Comparing Manual Therapy with the Use of Cold Packs in the Treatment of Post-Traumatic Headache." *Cephalalgia* 10, no. 5 (1990): 2241–50.

Ji, T., C. Lin, L. S. Krill, et al. "Flavokawain B, a Kava Chalcone, Inhibits Growth of Human Osteosarcoma Cells through G2/M Cell Cycle Arrest and Apoptosis." *Mol Cancer* 12 (2013): 55. doi: 10.1186/1476-4598-12-55.

Johansson, L., X. Guo, T. Hällström, M. C. Norton, M. Waern, S. Östling, C. Bengtsson, and I. Skoog. "Common Psychosocial Stressors in Middle-Aged Women Related to Longstanding Distress and Increased Risk of Alzheimer's Disease: A 38-Year Longitudinal Population Study." *BMJ Open* 3, no. 9 (2013). doi: 10.1136/bmj open-2013-003142.

Johnson, B. A. "Herbal Formulas Show Market Growth." *Herbalgram* 46 (1999): 57.

Jordan, C. S., and K. T. Lenington. "Physiological Correlates of Eidetic Imagery and Induced Anxiety." *J Mental Imagery* 3, no. 1–2 (Fall 1979): 31–42.

Kabat-Zinn, J., L. Lipworth, R. Burney, and W. Sellers. "Four-Year Follow-Up of a Meditation-Based Program for the Self-Regulation of Chronic Pain: Treatment Outcomes and Compliance." *Clin J Pain* 2 (1986): 159–73.

Kamenícek, V., P. Holán, and P. Franĕk. "Systemic Enzyme Therapy in the Treatment and Prevention of Post-Traumatic and Postoperative Swelling." *Acta Chir Orthop Traumatol Cech* 68, no. 1 (2001): 45–49.

Kanowski, S., W. M. Herrmann, K. Stephan, W. Wierich, and R. Hoerr. "Proof of Efficacy of the Ginkgo biloba Special Extract EGB 761 in Outpatients Suffering from Mild to Moderate Primary Degenerative Dementia of the Alzheimer Type or Multi-Infarct Dementia." *Pharmacopsychiatry* 29 (1996): 47–56.

Kaplan, K. H., D. L. Goldenberg, and M. G. Nadeau. "The Impact of a Meditation-Based Stress Reduction Program on Fibromyalgia." *Gen Hosp Psych* 15, no. 5 (1993): 284–89.

Keniger, L. E., K. J. Gaston, K. N. Irvine, and R. A. Fuller. "What Are the Benefits of Interacting with Nature?" *Int J Environ Res Public Health* 10, no. 3 (Mar 2013): 913–35. Published online Mar 6, 2013. doi: 10.3390/ijerph10030913. PMCID: PMC3709294.

Kerkhoffs, G. M., P. A. Struijs, C. de Wit, V. W. Rahlfs, H. Zwipp, and C. N. van Dijk. "A Double Blind, Randomized, Parallel Group Study on the Efficacy and Safety of Treating Acute Lateral Ankle Sprain with Oral Hydrolytic Anzymes." *Br J Sports Med* 38, no. 4 (Aug 2004): 431–35.

Khamba, B. K., M. Aucoin, D. Tsirgielis, et al. "Effectiveness of Vitamin D in the Treatment of Mood Disorders: A Literature Review." *J Orthomolecular Med* 26, no. 3 (2011).

Kim, S., H. J. Kim, J. S. Yeo, S. J. Hong, J. M. Lee, and Y. Jeon. "The Effect of Lavender Oil of Stress, Bispectral Index Values, and Needle Insertion Pain in Volunteers." *J Altern Complement Med* 17 (2011): 823–26.

Kim, Y. I. "Role of Folate in Colon Cancer Development and Progression." *J Nutr* 133, no. 11, suppl. 1 (Nov 2003): 3731S–39S.

Kimmatkar N., V. Thawani, L. Hingorani, and R. Khiyani. "Efficacy and Tolerability of Boswellia serrata Extract in Treatment of Osteoarthritis of Knee: A Randomized Double Blind Placebo Controlled Trial." *Phytomedicine* 10, no. 1 (2003): 3–7. www.ncbi.nlm.nih.gov/pubmed/12622457.

Kinney, C. K., D. M. Rogers, K. A. Nash, and C. O. Bray. "Holistic Healing for Women with Breast Cancer through a Mind, Body, and Spirit Self-Empowerment." *J Holistic Nurs* 21, no. 3 (Sep 2003): 260–79. doi: 10.1177/0898010103254919.

Kinzler, E., J. Kromer, and E. Lehmann. "Wirksamkeit Eines Kava-Spezial-Extraktes Bei Patienten Mit Angst-, Spannungs-Und Erregungszustanden Nicht-Psychotischer Genese." *Arzneimittelforschung* 41 (1991): 584–88.

Kleijnen, J., and P. Knipschild. "Ginkgo biloba." *Lancet* 340 (1992): 1136–39.

Ko, G. D., N. B. Nowacki, L. Arseneau, M. Eitel, and A. Hum. "Omega-3 Fatty Acids for Neuropathic Pain: Case Series." *Clin J Pain* 26, no. 2 (2010): 168–72. doi: 10.1097/AJP.0b013e3181bb8533.

Koenig, H. G. "Religion and Remission of Depression in Medical Inpatients with Heart Failure/Pulmonary Disease." *J Nervous Mental Dis* 195 (2007): 389–95.

Kokjohn, K., D. M. Schmid, J. J. Triano, and P. C. Brennan. "The Effect of Spinal Manipulation on Pain and Prostaglandin Levels in Women with Primary Dysmenorrhea." *J Manipulative Physiol Ther* 15, no. 5 (1992): 279–85.

Kolata, Gina. "Death Rates Rising for Middle-Aged White Americans, Study Finds." *New York Times,* Nov 2, 2015.

Kotchen, T. A. "Historical Trends and Milestones in Hypertension Research A Model of the Process of Translational Research." *Hypertension* 58 (2011): 522–38. Published online Aug 22, 2011. doi: 10.1161/HYPERTENSIONAHA.111.177766.

Kreiman, G., C. Koch, and I. Fried. "Imagery Neurons in the Human Brain." *Nature* 16, no. 408 (Nov 2000): 357–61.

Kuvalaynanda, Swami. "Oxygen Absorption and Carbon Dioxide Elimination in Pranayama." *Yoga-Mimamsa* 4, no. 2 (1930): 95120.

Lao, L., S. Bergman, G. R. Hamilton, P. Langenberg, and B. Berman. "Evaluation of Acupuncture for Pain Control after Oral Surgery: A Placebo-Controlled Trial." *Arch Otolaryngol Head Neck Surg* 125, no. 5 (1999): 567–72. doi:10.1001/archotol.125.5.567.

Lawless, Julia. *The Illustrated Encycolpedia of Essential Oils: The Complete Guide to the Use of Oils in Aromatherapy and Herbalism.* Rockport, Mass.: Element Books, 1995.

LeShan, Lawrence. *The Medium, the Mystic, and the Physicist.* New York: Viking, 1966.

Lewandowski, W. A. "Patterning of Pain and Power with Guided Imagery." *Nurs Sci Q* 17, no. 3 (Jul 2004): 233–41.

Lewit, K., and D. G. Simons. "Myofascial Pain: Relief by Post-Isometric Relaxation." *Arch Phys Med Rehabil* 65, no. 8 (Aug 1984): 452–56.

Lindahl, O., and L. Lindwall. "Double Blind Study of a Valerian Preparation." *Pharmacol Biochem Behav* 32 (1989): 1065–66.

Linde, K., G. Allais, B. Brinkhaus, et al. "Acupuncture for the Prevention of Episodic Migraine." *Cochrane Database Syst Rev* 28, no. 6 (Jun 2016): CD001218. doi: 10.1002/14651858.CD001218.pub3.

Lindfors, P., P. Unge, P. Arvidsson, et al. "Effects of Gut-Directed Hypnotherapy on IBS in Different Clinical Settings: Results from Two Randomized, Controlled Trials." *Amer J Gastroenter* 107, no. 2 (2011): 276. doi: 10.1038/ajg.2011.340.

Lindfors, P., P. Unge, H. Nyhlin, et al. "Long-Term Effects of Hypnotherapy in Patients with Refractory Irritable Bowel Syndrome." *Scandinavian J Gastroenter* 47, no. 4 (2012): 414. doi: 10.3109/00365521.2012.658858.

Little, P., L. Smith, T. Cantrell, J. Chapman, J. Langridge, and R. Pickering. "General Practitioners' Management of Acute Back Pain: A Survey of Reported Practice Compared with Clinical Guidelines." *Brit Med J* 312 (1996): 485–88.

Liu, C. Z., J. P. Xie, L. P. Wang, et al. "Immediate Analgesia Effect of a Single Point Acupuncture in Primary Dymenorrhea: A Randomized Controlled Trial." *Pain Med* 12, no. 2 (Feb 2011): 300–307. Epub Dec 17, 2010. doi: 10.1111/j.1526-4637.2010.01017.x. Erratum in *Pain Med* 12, no. 4 (Apr 2011): 685.

Logan, A. C. "Omega-3 Fatty Acids and Major Depression: A Primer for the Mental Health Professional." *Lipids Health Dis* 3 (2004): 25. Published online Nov 9, 2004. doi: 10.1186/1476-511X-3-25. PMCID: PMC53386.

Longworth, J. C. D. "Psychophysiological Effects of Slow Stroke Back Massage in Normotensive Females." *Adv Nurs Sci,* 4, no. 4 (July 1982): 44–61.

Lorenzetti, B. E., G. E. Souza, S. J. Sarti, et al. "Myrcene Mimics the Peripheral Analgesic Activity of Lemongrass Tea." *J Ethnopharmacol* 34, no. 1 (1991): 43–48.

Lowe, Whitney W. "Orthopedic Massage." In *Primal's 3D Human Anatomy for Massage and Manual Therapies,* edited by Judith Delany. London: Primal Pictures, 2012.

Luria, A. R. *The Mind of a Mnemonist: A Little Book about a Vast Memory.* Cambridge, Mass.: Harvard University Press, 1968.

Madison, A. S. "Psychophysiological Response of Female Nursing Home Residents to Back Massage: An Investigation of One Type of Touch." Doctoral thesis, University of Maryland, 1973.

Maizels, M., A. Blumenfeld, and R. Burchette. "A Combination of Riboflavin, Magnesium, and Feverfew for Migraine Prophylaxis: A Randomized Trial." *Headache* 44 (2004): 885–90.

Malouf, M., E. J. Grimley, and S. L. Areosa. "Folic Acid with or without Vitamin B12 for Cognition and Dementia." *Cochrane Database Syst Rev* 4 (2003): CD004514.

Manjunath, N. K., and S. Telles. "Influence of Yoga and Ayurveda on Self-Rated Sleep in a Geriatric Population." *Indian J Med Res* 121, no. 5 (May 2005): 683–90.

Martin, A., P. G. Schauble, S. H. Rai, and R. W. Curry Jr. "Effects of Hypnosis on the Labor Processes and Birth Outcomes of Pregnant Adolescents." *J Fam Practice* 50, no. 5 (May 2001): 441–43.

Matthews, D. A., S. M. Marlowe, and F. S. MacNutt. "Effects of Intercessory Prayer on Patients with Rheumatoid Arthritis." *Southern Med J* 93, no. 12 (2000): 1177–86.

Maury, Marguerite. *The Secret of Life and Youth.* London: Macdonald, 1964.

Mauskop, A., and B. M. Altura. "Role of Magnesium in the Pathogenesis and Treatment of Migraines." *Clin Neurosci* 5 (1998): 24–27.

Mauskop, A., B. T. Altura, and B. M. Altura. "Serum Ionized Magnesium Levels and Serum Ionized Calcium/Ionized Magnesium Ration in Women with Menstrual Migraine." *Headache* 42, no. 4 (2002): 242–48.

Mauskop, A., and J. J. Varughese. "Why All Migraine Patients Should Be Treated with Magnesium." *J Neural Transm* 119, no. 5 (May 2012): 575–79. Epub Mar 18, 2012. doi: 10.1007/s00702-012-0790-2.

Mayer, D. J., D. D. Price, and A. Rafii. "Antagonism of Acupuncture Analgesia in Man by the Narcotic Antagonist Naloxone." *Brain Res* 121, no. 2 (1977): 368.

McCown, Donald, and Marc Micozzi. "Mind-Body Thought and Practice." In *Fundamentals of Complementary and Alternative Medicine*, 5th ed., edited by Marc Micozzi, 70–87. Philadelphia: Elsevier Health Sciences, 2015.

———. *New World Mindfulness: From the Founding Fathers, Emerson, and Thoreau to Your Personal Practice.* Rochester, Vt.: Healing Arts Press, 2012.

McCown, Donald, Diane K. Reibel, and Marc Micozzi. *Teaching Mindfulness: A Practical Guide for Clinicians and Educators.* New York: Springer, 2011.

McCrory, D. C. *Evidence Report: Behavior and Physical Treatments for Tension-*

Type and Cervicogenic Headaches. Des Moines, Iowa: Foundation for Chiropractic Education and Research, 2001.

Mckechnie, A. A., F. Wilson, N. Watson, and D. Scott. "Anxiety States: A Preliminary Report on the Value of Connective Tissue Massage." *J Psychosom Res* 27, no. 2 (1983): 125.

Meade, T. W., S. Dyer, W. Browne, and A. O. Frank. "Randomised Comparison of Chiropractic and Hospital Outpatient Management for Low Back Pain: Results from Extended Follow Up." *Brit Med J* 311, no. 7001 (1995): 349–51.

Meeker, W., D. Lawrence, M. S. Micozzi, et al. "Consensus Development on Treatment of Lower Back Pain." Washington, D.C.: American Public Health Association, 2007.

Merolla, G., F. Dellabiancia, A. Ingardia, et al. "Co-Analgesic Therapy for Arthroscopic Supraspinatus Tendon Repair Pain Using a Dietary Supplement Containing Boswellia serrata and Curcuma longa: A Prospective Randomized Placebo-Controlled Study." *Musculoskelet Surg* 99, suppl. 1 (Sep 2015): S43–52.

Micozzi, Marc S. *Celestial Healing.* Philadelphia: Singing Dragon Press, 2011.

Miller, Light, and Bryan Miller. *Ayurveda and Aromatherapy: The Earth Essential Guide to Ancient Wisdom and Modern Healing.* Twin Lakes, Wisc.: Lotus Press, 1995.

Mills, N., and J. Allen. "Mindfulness of Movement as a Coping Strategy in Multiple Sclerosis: A Pilot Study." *Gen Hosp Psychiatry* 22, no. 6 (Nov–Dec 2000): 425–31.

Mishra, Lakshmi Chandra. *Rheumatoid Arthritis, Osteoarthritis, and Gout: Scientific Basis for Ayurvedic Therapies.* Boca Raton, Fla.: CRC Press, 2004.

Mishra, Lakshmi-Chandra, and Betsy B. Singh, "Scientific Basis for the Therapeutic Use of Withania somnifera (Ashwagandha): A Review." *Altern Med Rev* 5, no. 4 (2000).

Montgomery, G. H., D. David, G. Winkel, et al. "The Effectiveness of Adjunctive Hypnosis with Surgical Patients: A Meta-Analysis." *Anesth Analg* 94 (2002): 1639–45.

Montgomery, G. H., K. N. DuHamel, and W. H. Redd. "A Meta-Analysis of Hypnotically Induced Analgesia: How Effective Is Hypnosis?" *Int J Clin Exp Hypn* 48, no. 2 (2000): 138–53.

Morley, J. E. "Dementia: Does Vitamin D Modulate Cognition?" *Nature Rev Neurol* 10 (2014): 613–14. Published online Oct 21, 2014. doi:10.1038/nrneurol.2014.193.

Morris, Desmond. *The Human Zoo: A Zoologist's Study of the Urban Animal.* New York: Oxford University Press, 1995.

Morris, M. C., D. A. Evans, J. L. Bienias, et al. "Dietary Folate and Vitamin B12

Intake and Cognitive Decline among Community-Dwelling Older Persons." *Archives Neurol* 62, no. 4 (April 2005): 641–45.

Mueller, H. H., C. C. Donaldson, D. V. Nelson, and M. Layman. "Treatment of Fibromyalgia Incorporating EEG-Driven Stimulation: A Clinical Outcomes Study." *J Clin Psychol* 57, no. 7 (Jul 2001): 933–52.

Mulrow, C., V. Lawrence, R. Ackermann, et al. "Garlic: Effects on Cardiovascular Risks and Disease, Protective Effects against Cancer, and Clinical Adverse Effects: Summary. 2000 Oct." In *AHRQ Evidence Report Summaries*, 20. Rockville, Md.: Agency for Healthcare Research and Quality, 1998–2005. www.ncbi.nlm.nih.gov/books/NBK11910/.

Mynott, T. L., S. Guandalini, F. Raimondi, and A. Fasano. "Bromelain Prevents Secretion Caused by Vibrio cholerae and Escherichia coli Enterotoxins in Rabbit Ileum In Vitro." *Gastroentero* 113, no. 1 (1997): 175–84.

Nabi, H., M. Kivimäki, G. D. Batty, M. J. Shipley, A. Britton, E. J. Brunner, J. Vahtera, C. Lemogne, A. Elbaz, and A. Singh-Manoux. "Increased Risk of Coronary Heart Disease among Individuals Reporting Adverse Impact of Stress on Their Health: The Whitehall II Prospective Cohort Study." *Eur Heart J,* epub ahead of print, June 26, 2013.

Najafizade, N., S. Hemati, A. Gookizade, et al. "Preventive Effects of Zinc Sulfate on Taste Alterations in Patients under Irradiation for Head and Neck Cancers: A Randomized Placebo-Controlled Trial." *Arbab J Res Med Sci* 18, no. 2 (Feb 2013): 123–26. PMCID: PMC3724372.

Nelson, C. F., G. Bronfort, R. Evans, P. Boline, C. Goldsmith, and A. V. Anderson. "The Efficacy of Spinal Manipulation, Amitriptyline and the Combination of Both Therapies for the Prophylaxis of Migraine Headache." *J Manipulative Physiol Ther* 21, no. 8 (1998): 511–19.

O'Keeffe, S. T., K. Gavin, and J. N. Lavan. "Iron Status and Restless Legs Syndrome in the Elderly." *Age Ageing* 23 (1994): 200–203.

Oken, B. S., D. M. Storzbach, and J. A. Kaye. "The Efficacy of Ginkgo biloba on Cognitive Function in Alzheimer Disease." *Arch Neurol* 55 (1998): 1409–15.

Olness, K. N., and M. M. Conroy. "A Pilot Study of Voluntary Control of Transcutaneuos PO2 by Children: A Brief Communication." *Int J Clin Experimental Hypn* 33, no. 1 (1985): 1–5.

Olness, Karen, and G. Gail Gardner. *Hypnosis and Hypnotherapy with Children.* New York: Grune and Stratton, 1988.

Pargamont, K. I., H. G. Koenig, and L. M. Perez. "The Many Methods of Religious Coping: Development and Initial Validation of the RCOPE." *J Clin Psychol* 56, no. 4 (2000): 519–43.

Peanpadungrat, P. "Efficacy and Safety of Fish Oil in Treatment of Knee Osteoarthritis." *J Med Assoc Thai* 98, suppl. 3 (April 2015): S110–14

Pearce, Joseph Chilton. *Magical Child.* New York: Plume, 1977.

Peikert, A., C. Wilimzig, and R. Köhne-Volland. "Prophylaxis of Migraine with Oral Magnesium: Results from a Prospective, Multi-Center, Placebo-Controlled and Double-Blind Randomized Study." *Cephalalgia* 16 (1996): 257–63.

Pemberton, R. "The Physiology of Massage." In *American Medical Association Handbook of Physical Medicine and Rehabilitation.* Philadelphia, Pa.: American Medical Association, 1950.

Pericleous, M., D. Mandair, and M. E. Caplin. "Diet and Supplements and Their Impact on Colorectal Cancer." *J Gastrointest Oncol* 4, no. 4 (2013): 409–23. doi: 10.3978/j.issn.2078-6891.2013.003.

Perlman, S. "Dentistry." In *Medical Hypnosis: An Introduction and Clinical Guide,* edited by Roberta Temes, 131–39. New York: Churchill Livingstone, 1999.

Pfaffenrath, V., P. Wessely, C. Meyer, et al. "Magnesium in the Prophylaxis of Migraine: A Double-Blind, Placebo-Controlled Study." *Cephalalgia* 16 (1996): 436–40.

Pittler, M. H., and E. Ernst. "Efficacy of Kava Extract for Treating Anxiety: Systematic Review and Meta-Analysis." *J Clin Psychopharm* 20, no. 1 (Feb 2000): 84–89.

Pomeranz, B., and L. Bibic. "Electroacupuncture Suppresses a Nociceptive Reflex: Naltrexone Prevents but Does Not Reverse This Effect." *Brain Res* 452, no. 1–2 (June 1988): 27–31.

Pomeranz, B., and D. Chiu. "Naloxone Blockade of Acupuncture Analgesia: Endorphin Implicated." *Life Sci* 19 (1976): 1757–62.

Prentiss, Karen Pechilis. *The Embodiment of Bhakti.* Oxford: Oxford University, 1999.

Rahman, K., and G. M. Lowe. "Aged Garlic Extract Reduces Low Attenuation Plaque in Coronary Arteries of Patients with Metabolic Syndrome in a Prospective Randomized Double-Blind Study." *J Nutr* 146 (2016): 427S–32S.

Ricci, Jeanne. "T.K.V. Desikachar Developed Viniyoga to Fit Each Individual Student." *Yoga Journal,* Aug 28, 2007.

Richard, L., R. L. Nahin, P. M. Barnes, and B. J. Stussman. "Expenditures on Complementary Health Approaches: United States, 2012." *National Health Statistics Reports* 95 (June 22, 2016).

Richards, K. C., R. Gibson, and L. Overton-McCoy. "Effects of Massage in Acute and Critical Care." *AACN Clin Issues: Adv Prac Acute and Critical Care* 11 (2000): 77–96.

Riddle, D. L., W. A. Jiranek, and C. W. Hayes. "Use of a Validated Algorithm to Judge the Appropriateness of Total Knee Arthroplasty in the United States: A Multicenter Longitudinal Cohort Study." *Arthrit Rheumat* 66 (2014): 2134–43. doi:10.1002/art.38685.

Rivlin, R. S. "Magnesium Deficiency and Alcohol Intake: Mechanisms, Clinical Significance, and Possible Relation to Cancer Development (A Review)." *J Am Coll Nutr* 13 (1994): 416–23.

Robinson, J. G., N. Ijioma, and W. Harris. "Omega-3 Fatty Acids and Cognitive Function in Women." *Women's Health* (London, England) 6, no. 1 (2010): 119–34. doi: 10.2217/whe.09.75.

Rod, K. "Observing the Effects of Mindfulness-Based Meditation on Anxiety and Depression in Chronic Pain Patients." *Psychiat Danub* 27, suppl. 1 (Sep 2015): S209–11.

Rogovik, A. L., and R. D. Goldman. "Hypnosis for Treatment of Pain in Children." *Can Fam Physician* 53, no. 5 (2007): 823–25.

Rosenstein, D. L., R. J. Elin, J. M. Hosseini, et al. "Magnesium Measures across the Menstrual Cycle in Premenopausal Syndrome." *Biol Psychiat* 35 (1994): 557–61.

Rubin, G. "A New Bromelain-Based Enzyme for the Release of Dupuytren's Contracture: Dupuytren's Enzymatic Bromelain-Based Release." *Bone Joint Res* 5 (2016): 175–77. doi: 10.1302/2046-3758.55.BJR-2016-0072.

Sacks, M. H. "Exercise for Stress Control." In *Mind-Body Medicine: How to Use Your Mind for Better Health,* edited by David Goleman and Joel Gunn, 233–57. Yonkers, N.Y.: Consumer Reports, 1998.

Schwartz, Nancy M., and Mark S. Schwartz. "Definitions of Biofeedback and Applied Psychophysiology." In *Biofeedback: A Practitioners Guide*, 3rd ed., edited by Mark S. Schwartz and Frank Andrasik, 128–58. New York: Guilford Press, 2003.

Segerdahl, A. R., M. Mezue, T. W. Okell, J. T. Farrar, and I. Tracey. "The Dorsal Posterior Insula Subserves a Fundamental Role in Human Pain." *Nature Neuroscience* 18 (2015): 499–500. www.nature.com/neuro/journal/v18/n4/full/nn.3969.html.

Selye, Hans. *The Stress of Life.* New York: McGraw-Hill, 1978.

Shah, Pravin K., ed. "Jain Fundamentals, Jain Rituals, Jain Scriptures, Jain Compassion, Compassionate Quotes." Jain Study Center of North Carolina. www.fas.harvard.edu/~pluralsm/affiliates/jainism/workshop/Pathashal%20Workshop98.PDF.

Shekelle, P. G., I. Coulter, E. L. Hurwitz, et al. "Congruence between Decisions to Initiate Chiropractic Spinal Manipulation for Low Back Pain and Appropriateness Criteria in North America." *Ann Intern Med* 129, no. 1 (1998): 9–17.

Shepherd, Gordon M. *Neurobiology.* Oxford: Oxford University Press, 1983.

Sherwood, R. A., B. F. Rocks, A. Steward, et al. "Magnesium and Premenstrual Syndrome." *Ann Clin Biochem* 23 (1986): 667–70.

Shils, Maurice E. "Nutrition and Diet in Cancer Management." In *Modern*

Nutrition in Health and Disease, 9th ed., edited by Maurice E. Shils, James A. Olson, Moshe Shihe, and A. Catharine Ross, 1317–47. Baltimore, Md.: Williams and Wilkins, 1999.

Singh, U., and I. Jialal. "Alpha-Lipoic Acid Supplementation and Diabetes." *Nutr Rev* 66, no. 11 (2008): 646–57.

Sloman, R. "Relaxation and Imagery for Anxiety and Depression Control in Community Patients with Advanced Cancer." *Cancer Nurs* 25, no. 6 (Dec 2002): 432–35.

Smedby, K. M., H. Henrik, A. Mads Melbye, et al. "Ultraviolet Radiation Exposure and Risk of Malignant Lymphomas." *JNCI J Natl Cancer Inst* 97, no. 3 (2005): 199–209. doi: 10.1093/jnci/dji022.

Smith, C. A., C. T. Collins, A. M. Cyna, and C. A. Crowther. "Complementary and Alternative Therapies for Pain Management in Labour (Cochrane Review)." *Thecochrane Library* 3 (2004).

Solfvin, J. "Mental Healing." In *Advances in Parapsychological Research,* edited by Stanley Krippner, 31–63. Jefferson, N.C.: McFarland, 1984.

Spiegel, D. "The Mind Prepared: Hypnosis in Surgery." *J Nat Cancer Inst* 99 (2007): 1280–81.

Staples, Julie K. "Yoga." In *Fundamentals of Complementary and Alternative Medicine,* 5th ed., edited by Marc S. Micozzi, 332–43. St. Louis, Mo.: Elsevier, 2015.

Steele, J. J. "The Anthropology of Smell and Scent in Ancient Egypt and South American Shamanism." In *Fragrance: The Psychology and Biology of Perfume,* edited by S. Van Toller and G. H. Dodd. Barking, England: Elsevier Science Pub., 1992.

Stellar, J. E., N. John-Henderson, C. L. Anderson, A. M. Gordon, G. D. McNeil, and D. Keltner. "Positive Effect and Markers of Inflammation: Discrete Positive Emotions Predict Lower Levels of Inflammatory Cytokines." *Emotion* 15, no. 2 (Apr. 2015): 129–33. doi: 10.1037/emo0000033. Epub ahead of print Jan 19, 2015.

Stevensen, C. J. "The Psychophysiological Effects of Aromatherapy Massage following Cardiac Surgery." *Comple Ther Med* 2 (1994): 27–35.

Stoddart, D. M. "Human Odour Culture: A Zoological Perspective." In *Perfumery: The Psychology and Biology of Fragrance,* edited by Steve Van Toller and George H. Dodd, 3–18. London: Chapman and Hall, 1991.

Swaminathan, R. "Hypo-Hypermagnesaemia." In *Oxford Textbook of Nephrology,* 2nd ed., edited by A. M. Davison, J. S. Cameron, J. P. Gunfield, D. N. S. Kerr, and E. Ritz, 271–310. Oxford: Oxford University Press, 1998.

Targ, E. F., and E. G. Levine. "The Efficacy of a Mind-Body-Spirit Group for Women with Breast Cancer: A Randomized Controlled Trial." *Gen Hosp Psychiat* 24, no. 4 (Jul–Aug 2002): 238–48.

Thorgrimsen, L., A. Spector, A. Wiles, and M. Orrell. "Aromatherapy for Dementia (Cochrane Review)." *Thecochrane Library* 3 (2004).

Tillu, D. V., O. K. Melemedjian, M. N. Asiedu, et al. "Resveratrol Engages AMPK to Attenuate ERK and mTOR Signaling in Sensory Neurons and Inhibits Incision-Induced Acute and Chronic Pain." *Mol Pain* 8 (Jan 2012): 5. doi: 10.1186/1744-8069-8-5.

Tisserand, Robert. *The Art of Aromatherapy.* Saffron Waldon, England: Daniel Co. Ltd, 1988.

Tisserand, Robert, and Tony Balacs. *Essential Oil Safety: A Guide for Health Professionals.* Edinburgh: Churchill Livingstone, 1995.

Tisserand, Robert, and Rodney Young. *Essential Oil Safety.* 2nd ed. Edinburgh: Churchill Livingstone, 1995.

Toblin, R. L., P. J. Quartana, L. A. Riviere, K. C. Walper, and C. W. Hoge. "Chronic Pain and Opioid Use in U.S. Soldiers after Combat Deployment." *J Am Med Assoc Intern Med* 174, no. 8 (2014): 1400–401.

Torii, S., H. Fukuda, H. Kanemoto, R. Miyanchi, Y. Jamauzu, and M. Kawasaki. "Contingent Negative Variation (CNV) and the Psychological Effects of Odour." In *Perfumery: The Psychology and Biology of Fragrance,* edited by Steve Van Toller and George H. Dodd, 107–21. London: Chapman and Hall, 1988.

Toscano, W. B., and P. S. Cowlings. "Reducing Motion Sickness: A Comparison of Autogenic-Feedback Training and an Alternative Cognitive Task." *Aviat Space Environ Med* 53, no. 5 (1982): 449–53.

Tuchin, P. J., H. Pollard, and R. Bonello. "A Randomized Controlled Trial of Chiropractic Spinal Manipulative Therapy for Migraine." *J Manipulative Physiol Ther* 23, no. 2 (2000): 91–95.

Tupe, R. P., and S. A. Chiplonkar. "Zinc Supplementation Improved Cognitive Performance and Taste Acuity in Indian Adolescent Girls." *J Am Coll Nutr* 28, no. 4 (Aug 2009): 388–96.

Turk, A., and O. Ratkolb. "Mobilization of the Cervical Spine in Chronic Headaches." *Manual Med* 3 (1987): 15–17.

Tusek, D., J. M. Church, and V. W. Fazio. "Guided Imagery as a Coping Strategy for Perioperative Patients." *AORN J* 66, no. 4 (Oct 1997): 644–49.

Tütüncü, N. B., M. Bayraktar, and K. Varli. "Reversal of Defective Nerve Conduction with Vitamin E Supplementation in Type 2 Diabetes: A Preliminary Study." *Diabetes Care* 21 (1998): 1915–18.

University of Wisconsin School of Medicine and Public Health. "Achieving Balance in Federal and State Pain Policy: A Guide to Evaluation" *Pain Policy and Studies Group* 2013. www.painpolicy.wisc.edu/sites/www.painpolicy .wisc.edu/files/evalguide2013.pdf.

University of Wisconsin School of Medicine and Public Health. "Achieving

Balance in State Pain Policy: A Progress Report Card." *Pain Policy and Studies Group* 2014. www.painpolicy.wisc.edu/sites/www.painpolicy.wisc .edu/files/prc2013.pdf.

Valnet, Jean. *The Practice of Aromatherapy.* Saffron Walden, England: Daniel Co., 1990.

Vamvakas, S., M. Teschner, U. Bahner, and A. Heidland. "Alcohol Abuse: Potential Role in Electrolyte Disturbances and Kidney Diseases." *Clin Nephrol* 49 (1998): 205–13.

Van Dongen, M., E. van Rossum, A. Kessels, H. Sielhorst, and P. Knipschild. "Ginkgo for Elderly People with Dementia and Age-Associated Memory Impairment: A Randomized Clinical Trial." *J Clin Epidemiol* 56, no. 4 (2003): 367–76.

Vernon, H., K. Humphreys, and C. Hagino. "Chronic Mechanical Neck Pain in Adults Treated by Manual Therapy: A Systematic Review of Change Scores in Randomized Clinical Trials." *J Manipulative Physiol Ther* 30, no. 3 (2007): 215–27.

Veugelers, P. J., and J. P. Ekwaru. "A Statistical Error in the Estimation of the Recommended Dietary Allowance for Vitamin D." *Nutrients* 6, no. 10 (Oct 2014): 4472–75. Published online Oct 20, 2014. doi: 10.3390/ nu6104472. PMCID: PMC4210929.

Vincent, C. A. "A Controlled Trial of the Treatment of Migraine by Acupuncture." *Clin J Pain* 5, no. 4 (Dec 1989): 305–12.

Volz, H. P., and M. Kieser. "Kava-Kava Extract WS 1490 versus Placebo in Anxiety Disorders: A Randomized Placebo-Controlled 25-Week Outpatient Trial." *Pharmacopsychiatry* 30 (1997): 1–5.

Von Boetticher, A. "Ginkgo biloba Extract in the Treatment of Tinnitus: A Systemic Review." *Neuropsychiat Dis Treat* 7 (2011): 441–47. doi: 10.2147/ NDT.S22793.

Wang, F., S. K. Van Den Eeden, L. M. Ackerson, S. E. Salk, R. H. Reince, and R. J. Elin. "Oral Magnesium Oxide Prophylaxis of Frequent Migrainous Headache in Children: A Randomized, Double-Blind, Placebo-Controlled Trial." *Headache* 43, no. 6 (2003): 601–10.

Weinmann, S., S. Roll, C. Schwarzbach, C. Vauth, and S. N. Willich. "Effects of Ginkgo biloba in Dementia: Systematic Review and Meta-Analysis." *BMC Geriatr* 10 (2010): 14. Published online Mar 17, 2010. doi: 10.1186/1471-2318-10-14.

Welge-Lüssen, A. "Re-Establishment of Olfactory and Taste Functions." *GMS Curr Top Otorhinolaryngol Head Neck Surg* 4 (2005): Doc06. Epub Sep 28 2005.

Wells, N., C. Pasero, and M. McCaffery. "Improving the Quality of Care through Pain Assessment and Management." Chapter 17 in *Patient Safety and Quality: An Evidence-Based Handbook for Nurses,* edited by Ronda G. Hughes. Rockville, Md.: Agency for Healthcare Research and Quality, Apr 2008. www.ncbi.nlm.nih.gov/books/NBK2658/.

White, K. D. "Salivation: The Significance of Imagery in Its Voluntary Control." *Psychophysiol* 15 (1978): 196–203. doi:10.1111/j.1469-8986.1978.tb01363.x.

Wilber, K. "Psychologic Perennis: The Spectrum of Consciousness." *J Transpersonal Psychol* 7, no. 2 (1975): 111.

Wilk v. American Medical Association, 671 F. Supp. 1465 (N.D. Ill. 1987).

Wilkins, C. H., Y. I. Sheline, C. M. Roe, S. J. Birge, and J. C. Morris. "Vitamin D Deficiency Is Associated with Low Mood and Worse Cognitive Performance in Older Adults." *Am J Geriatr Psychiat* 14, no. 12 (Dec 2006): 1032–40.

Wilkinson, S., J. Aldridge, I. Salmon, E. Cain, and B. Wilson. "An Evaluation of Aromatherapy Massage in Palliative Care." *Palliat Med* 13, no. 5 (Sep 1999): 409–17.

Williams, D. "Lecture Notes on Essential Oils." London: Eve Taylor Ltd., 1989.

Wilson, M. L., and P. A. Murphy. "Herbal and Dietary Therapies for Primary and Secondary Dysmenorrhoea." *The Cochrane Library* 2 (2002).

Winters, J. C., J. S. Sobel, K. H. Groenier, H. J. Arendzen, and B. Meyboom-de Jong. "Comparison of Physiotherapy, Manipulation, and Corticosteroid Injection for Treating Shoulder Complaints in General Practice: Randomised, Single Blind Study." *Brit Med J* 314, no. 7090 (1997): 1320–25.

Woodyard, C. "Exploring the Therapeutic Effects of Yoga and Its Ability to Increase Quality of Life." *Int J Yoga* 4, no. 2 (Jul–Dec 2011): 49–54. doi: 10.4103/0973-6131.85485. PMCID: PMC3193654.

Yagi, T., A. Asakawa, H. Ueda, S. Ikeda, S. Miyawaki, and A. Inui. "The Role of Zinc in the Treatment of Taste Disorders." *Recent Pat Food Nutr Agric* 5, no. 1 (Apr 2013): 44–51.

Yazici, Z. M., I. Sayin, G. Gökkuş, E. Alatas, H. Kaya, and F. T. Kayhan. "Effectiveness of Ericksonian Hypnosis in Tinnitus Therapy: Preliminary Results." *B-Ent* 8, no. 1 (2012): 7–12. www.ncbi.nlm.nih.gov/pubmed/22545384.

Ziegler, D., and F. A. Gries. "Alpha-Lipoic Acid in the Treatment of Diabetic Peripheral and Cardiac Autonomic Neuropathy." *Diabetes* 46, suppl 2 (1997): S62–66.

Index